VOLUME FIFTY FOUR

INTERNATIONAL REVIEW OF RESEARCH IN DEVELOPMENTAL DISABILITIES

Service Delivery Systems for Individuals with Intellectual and Developmental Disabilities and their Families Across the Lifespan

VOLUME FIFTY FOUR

INTERNATIONAL REVIEW OF RESEARCH IN DEVELOPMENTAL DISABILITIES

Service Delivery Systems for Individuals with Intellectual and Developmental Disabilities and their Families Across the Lifespan

Edited by

MEGHAN M. BURKE
University of Illinois at Urbana-Champaign, Champaign, IL, United States

ELSEVIER

ACADEMIC PRESS
An imprint of Elsevier

Academic Press is an imprint of Elsevier
125 London Wall, London EC2Y 5AS, United Kingdom
525 B Street, Suite 1650, San Diego, CA 92101, United States
50 Hampshire Street, 5th Floor, Cambridge, MA 02139, United States
The Boulevard, Langford Lane, Kidlington, Oxford OX5 1GB, United Kingdom

First edition 2018

ISBN: 978-0-12-815091-7
ISSN: 2211-6095

Publisher: Zoe Kruze
Acquisition Editor: Sam Mahfoudh
Editorial Project Manager: Teresa Pons-Ferrer
Production Project Manager: Abdulla Sait
Cover Designer: Victoria Pearson

Typeset by TNQ Technologies

CONTENTS

CONTRIBUTORS

Nicole B. Adams
University of Illinois, Urbana-Champaign, IL, United States

Heather M. Aldersey
Queen's University, Kingston, ON, Canada

Brian A. Boyd
Juniper Gardens Children's Project, University of Kansas, Kansas City, KS, United States

Meghan M. Burke
University of Illinois at Urbana-Champaign, Champaign, IL, United States

Marie Moore Channell
University of Illinois at Urbana-Champaign, Champaign, IL, United States

Grace L. Francis
George Mason University, Fairfax, VA, United States

Kami Gallus
Oklahoma State University, Stillwater, OK, United States

Bridgette L. Garcia
Vanderbilt Kennedy Center UCEDD, Nashville, TN, United States; Department of Special Education, Peabody College, Vanderbilt University, Nashville, TN, United States

George S. Gotto
University of Missouri at Kansas City - Institute for Human Development, Kansas City, MO, United States

Judith M.S. Gross
Indiana University, Bloomington, IN, United States

Shana J. Haines
University of Vermont, Burlington, VT, United States

Megan Hart
Vanderbilt Kennedy Center UCEDD, Nashville, TN, United States

Robert M. Hodapp
Vanderbilt Kennedy Center UCEDD, Nashville, TN, United States; Department of Special Education, Peabody College, Vanderbilt University, Nashville, TN, United States

Iheoma U. Iruka
HighScope Educational Research Foundation, Ypsilanti, MI, United States

Jennifer Jones
Oklahoma State University, Stillwater, OK, United States

Kathleen B. Kyzar
Texas Christian University, Fort Worth, TX, United States

Susan J. Loveall
University of Mississippi, 301 George Hall, University, MS, United States

Amie Lulinski
Coleman Institute for Cognitive Disabilities, Boulder, CO, United States

Louise Magiera
Indiana University, Bloomington, IN, United States

Elise McMillan
Vanderbilt Kennedy Center UCEDD, Nashville, TN, United States

Sophie A. Meskis
Vanderbilt Kennedy Center UCEDD, Nashville, TN, United States; Department of Special Education, Peabody College, Vanderbilt University, Nashville, TN, United States

Amalia Monroe-Gulick
University of Kansas, Lawrence, KS, United States

Susan B. Palmer
Beach Center on Disability, KUCDD, University of Kansas, Lawrence, KS, United States

Nigel P. Pierce
North Carolina Central University, Durham, NC, United States

Sascha Reed
George Mason University, Fairfax, VA, United States

Michelle C. Reynolds
University of Missouri at Kansas City - Institute for Human Development, Kansas City, MO, United States

Jan Rosemergy
Vanderbilt Kennedy Center UCEDD, Nashville, TN, United States

Joan Schmalzried
Indiana University, Bloomington, IN, United States

PREFACE

This special issue, the 54th issue of the *International Review of Research in Developmental Disabilities*, examines how families navigate service delivery systems across the life span. For individuals with intellectual and developmental disabilities (IDD), services range in relation to both the needs of the individuals with IDD and their ages. For children aged 0–3 years with IDD, services can include medical diagnostics (e.g., receiving a diagnosis) and educational supports (e.g., early intervention services). For 3- to 21-year-olds with IDD, although services vary, the school is often the primary provider of services and supports. Within school services, the emphasis shifts from the family to the individual with IDD. This shift is especially noticeable among transition-aged youth with IDD (i.e., individuals aged 14–22). Among this age range, the school system focuses on transition services to ensure positive postschool outcomes with respect to employment, independent living, education, and training. Finally, individuals aged 22 years and older may seek formal services and informal supports. Regarding the former, the adult service delivery system is fragmented and, unfortunately, often unable to support all adults with IDD. Perhaps as a result, individuals with IDD and their families often create natural, informal supports to fill this void.

In this special issue, the authors describe the service delivery system in relation to each of these age ranges. Specifically, they describe the current state of the literature as well as implications for future research, policy, and practice. Notably, the study of service delivery systems and their impact on individuals with IDD and their families is tedious. Every individual with IDD needs different supports and services in relation to their needs and strengths. Furthermore, service delivery systems vary with respect to federal, state, and local policies as well as in relation to the availability of resources. Thus, these authors should be applauded for venturing into this research given its inherently complex nature.

In the first manuscript, Brian Boyd and his colleagues (Iheoma Iruka and Nigel Pierce) propose a model and research agenda to address service disparities among families of children with autism spectrum disorder (ASD). Specifically, they describe the Behavioral Model of Health Service Use. Then, they adapt the model to describe its potential use to examine educational service disparities among families of color of children with ASD.

The research about service disparities clearly documents the need for a guiding conceptual framework; Dr. Boyd and has colleagues respond to this call with their adapted model. This manuscript has clear implications for future research about service disparities.

In the second manuscript, Shana Haines, Grace Francis, Kathleen Kyzar, Heather Aldersey, and Nicole Adams discuss family–professional partnerships among refugee families of children with disabilities. This manuscript beautifully articulates the systemic challenges among refugee families of children with disabilities in accessing needed school services. In their systematic literature review about refugee families of children with disabilities, Shana Haines and colleagues demonstrate the dearth of research among this population. Furthermore, they document the widespread barriers to accessing services. Their manuscript has important implications not only for future research but also for practice and policy.

Grace Francis, Judith Gross, Louise Magiera, Joan Schmalzried, Amalia Monroe-Gulick, and Sascha Reed then review the transition planning process for young adults with IDD. In their manuscript, they describe theory, policy, and researched programs and activities to improve transition planning. By dovetailing theory, policy, and programs, they provide a holistic understanding of transition planning including the supports available as well as the challenges in conducting high-quality transition planning. Their rich description of the landscape of transition planning then leads to fruitful implications for practice and research.

Marie Channell and Susan Loveall dive deeper into transition planning among a subpopulation—youth with Down syndrome. Using a phenotypic approach, they summarize the literature about postschool outcomes for young adults with Down syndrome. Based on gaps in the literature and the dismal outcomes for many young adults with Down syndrome, they offer suggestions for service delivery models as well as future research. Indeed, Marie and Susan offer a rare, etiology-driven approach to examine transition outcomes. More research would benefit from using a similar approach with other groups of individuals with specific types of disabilities (e.g., Williams syndrome, Prader–Willi syndrome).

Shifting focus from school to adult services, the next manuscript examines the current state of formal adult services for individuals with IDD. Specifically, Meghan Burke, Amie Lulinski, Jennifer Jones, and Kami Gallus review the history of adult services for individuals with IDD within the United States. Then, they describe the current state of the adult service delivery system along with pressing issues and decisions about the future of the service delivery system. Unlike school services, adult services are fragmented. Thus, this manuscript provides a glimpse into the complexity of adult services—an important but difficult to navigate system of services.

Perhaps because of the inadequacy of the adult service delivery system to meet the needs of all individuals with IDD, families often turn to natural or informal supports. Michelle Reynolds, Susan Palmer, and George Gotto eloquently describe natural supports in their manuscript. Specifically, they share the history of and context for natural supports as well as describe the LifeCourse Framework for integrated supports. Concluding with directions for future research about integrated supports, Michelle, Susan, and George provide important next steps for future research about services emphasizing that such research needs to include natural supports as well as individuals who do not currently receive formal support services.

In the final manuscript, Robert Hodapp, Jan Rosemergy, Bridgette Garcia, Sophie Meskis, Megan Hart, and Elise McMillan describe information and referral services for individuals with IDD and their families. Wrapping up this special issue, they describe services that are needed across the life span; thus, this manuscript relates to each of the previous manuscripts regardless of the age of the individual with IDD. An understudied but important resource for families, information, and referral services vary widely across the United States. This manuscript demonstrates the ways in which such services vary as well as needed research to examine the effectiveness of information and referral services.

Altogether, this special issue provides important reviews of the literature as well as next steps for future research, policy, and practice with respect to service delivery systems for individuals with IDD. When individuals with IDD and their families receive appropriate services and supports, they have better outcomes. Thus, it is critical that we continue to conduct research in this area. I thank each of the authors for contributing their expertise to this special issue. Also, I thank the reviewers for sharing their insights with the authors. Furthermore, I thank Drs. Robert Hodapp and Debbie Fidler for inviting me to be a guest editor. Finally, I thank Charlotte Rowley and Indhumathie Mani at Elsevier press. I hope you enjoy this special issue.

CHAPTER ONE

Strengthening Service Access for Children of Color With Autism Spectrum Disorders: A Proposed Conceptual Framework

Brian A. Boyd[*,1], **Iheoma U. Iruka**[§] **and Nigel P. Pierce**[¶]
[*]Juniper Gardens Children's Project, University of Kansas, Kansas City, KS, United States
[§]HighScope Educational Research Foundation, Ypsilanti, MI, United States
[¶]North Carolina Central University, Durham, NC, United States
[1]Corresponding Author: Email: brian.boyd@ku.edu

Contents

Abstract

Racial/ethnic minority and poor children with autism spectrum disorders seem to be at increased risk for poorer outcomes in comparison to their White, more affluent peers. Worse outcomes may occur for these children because they get access to lower quality and less effective services. In other fields, including medicine and public health,

International Review of Research in Developmental Disabilities, Volume 54
ISSN 2211-6095
https://doi.org/10.1016/bs.irrdd.2018.07.001

conceptual frameworks have been put forth and validated in order to identify barriers to healthcare access and utilization. We build upon such prior conceptual frameworks in order to the propose the *Model of School-Based Service Access for Children of Color with Autism Spectrum Disorders*. The goal is for this model to guide future research aimed at understanding why disparities in access to school-based services exist for this group, with the ultimate goal of eliminating those disparities.

1. INTRODUCTION

Racial/ethnic minority and poor children with autism spectrum disorder (ASD) continue to be diagnosed at later ages (Durkin et al., 2010; Mandell, Listerud, Levy, Pinto-Martin, 2002; Mandell et al., 2009), even though poverty may place children at increased risk of having the disorder (Rai et al., 2012). This creates disparities in early receipt of critical mental health and educational services that may slow or prevent the long-term consequences of the disorder. Even after receiving a diagnosis of ASD, minority and/or children from low-income families still are at risk for a host of poorer outcomes in comparison to their White peers including: more severe language delays (Tek & Landa, 2012), increased symptom severity (Blacher, Cohen, & Azad, 2014), receipt of lower quality or fewer services (Liptak et al., 2008; Magaña, Parish, Rose, Timberlake & Swaine, 2012; Thomas, Ellis, McLaurin, Daniels & Morrisey, 2007), and more difficulty accessing any services post high school (Shattuck, Wagner, Narendorf, Sterzing, & Hensley, 2011).

There is also evidence that parent socioeconomic status (SES) and demographic factors affect the positive outcomes of children with ASD. Fountain et al. (2012), using an extant database of approximately 7000 children from California, reported that children with ASD identified as "high functioning" (i.e., higher cognitive ability) were more likely to have non-Hispanic, White and well-educated mothers; whereas, racial minority children with less formally educated mothers were unlikely to experience symptom improvement over time. Similarly, Mehta, Lee, and Ylitalo (2013) used data from used the 1998 and 2009 waves of the National Health Interview Survey (NHIS), an annual and ongoing cross-sectional survey of the US non-institutionalized population to examine rates of ASD diagnosis across ethnic groups. They found the following: ASD diagnosis had an average annual increase in the odds of approximately 14%, with an increase of 15% for White children, but only 5% for Black children, in comparison to White children, there were no White-Asian or White-Hispanic differences in the trend. The authors signal this may be an indication of Black children with ASD potentially not being diagnosed or misdiagnosed, which could contribute to later receipt of services and poorer outcomes.

1.1 Relationship Between Ethnicity and Socioeconomic Status

Ethnicity and socioeconomic status (SES) are often confounded in US society. Ethnic minorities, specifically Black and Hispanic children are likely to be from low-resourced households compared to their White and Asian peers. The National Center for Children in Poverty reported that over 60% of American Indian, Black, and Hispanic children are living in low-income households compared to about 30% of White and Asian children (Jiang, Granja, & Korball, 2017). In fact, a report from the National Center for Education Statistics (Aud, Fox, & KewalRamani, 2010) consistently found that ethnic minority children, especially Black and Hispanic children were likely to be from single, female-headed households, live in poverty, have less educated mothers, and be in high-poverty communities. Additionally, low-income and ethnic minorities are also more likely to live in racially-segregated enclaves that are low-resourced with less abundant supply of high quality services and practitioners (Meyers & Jordan, 2006).

This confound between SES and ethnicity has implications for children's well-being and outcomes. Though still difficult to disentangle, studies are beginning to understand how SES and race/ethnicity may have unique and intersectional impacts on children's development. For example, the family investment model posits that SES, in the way of income, education, and time, provides the economic stability and knowledge base for families to purchase high quality enriching materials and services and ways to effectively implement and extend learning opportunities for the betterment of their children (Dodge, Bai, Ladd, & Muschkin, 2017; Haveman & Wolfe, 1995; Mistry, Biesanz, Chien, Howes, & Benner, 2008). A deeper analysis by scholars such as Raver, Gershoff, and Aber (2007) Iruka, LaForett, and Odom (2012), and Iruka, Dotterer and Pungello (2014) indicate that while this general notion is true, it does not function equivalently across ethnic groups. For example, in their study, Iruka et al. (2012) examined the family investment model across four ethnic groups — European Americans, African Americans, Hispanics, and Asians using a large nationally-representative data set. They found that the pathway between sociodemographic factors (e.g., SES, household structure, employment status) to children's language and numeracy through parent–child activities (e.g., reading, talking, singing) was only significant for European Americans; this pathway was not significant for other groups. Rather, the pathway from sociodemographic factors, including SES, to children's language and numeracy through parental sensitivity was most salient for European Americans, African Americans, and Spanish-speaking Hispanics; these models were not salient for Asians or English-speaking Hispanics.

1.2 Factors Linking Ethnicity and SES for Children With ASD

The most pervasive factors found linking ethnicity to outcomes are issues of racial and socioeconomic school segregation (Rumberger & Palardy, 2005), inequitable resource distribution (Greenwald, Hedges & Laine, 1996), and the disproportionate placement of underprepared teachers in high-poverty schools (Borman & Kimball, 2005; Darling-Hammond, 2004). Reardon and Fahle (2017) note that Black and Hispanic children are likely to live in poor communities, resulting in attendance in schools with greater concentration of poverty and disadvantage. These "high-poverty schools typically have fewer resources, poorer facilities, a harder time attracting and retaining skilled teachers, and more students in need of remediation and additional services. In addition, high-poverty schools typically have fewer students whose parents have economic, social, and political resources to invest in schools" (Reardon & Fahle, 2017, p. 21). In their review of New York City Elementary Schools, New York Appleseed (n.d.), a social just center that advocates for equity of access, found that after accounting for teacher experience, schools with a majority of Black, Latino, or non-White students had higher percentages of less qualified teachers than did schools with a majority of White students, as indicated by degree, teaching certificate, and turnover. Thus, concentrated disadvantage, primarily due to historical housing patterns are more likely experienced by children of color and have implications for children's well-being and quality of education, which are strongly related to the achievement gap.

Beyond issues of concentrated disadvantage, issues of race and ethnicity, regardless of income, also have an impact on children's outcomes. For example, in early childhood settings, issues of implicit bias and differential treatment have been noted. The US Department of Education Office for Civil Rights found in their 2013–14 Civil Rights Data Collection that Black public preschool children are 3.6 times more likely to receive one or more out-of-school suspensions as White preschool children, especially when Black children represent only 19% of preschool enrollment, but

47% of preschool children receiving one or more out-of-school suspensions; in comparison, White children represent 41% of preschool enrollment, but 28% of preschool children receiving one or more out-of-school suspensions. Furthermore, this same report also found disproportionality in regards to race/ethnicity and disability status in the K-12 system. Specifically, over 20% of American Indian, Native Hawaiian, Black, and multiracial boys with disabilities served by IDEA received one or more out-of-school suspensions compared to 10% of White boys with disabilities served by IDEA.

This issue of bias has also been supported in studies examining disproportionality in diagnosis and receipt of services for minority children. For example, Mehta et al. (2013) found evidence that the rate of diagnosis for Black children decreased between 1998 and 2009 and conjecture that it is not likely due to lower rates of ASD in Black children, regardless of SES, but the biases held by clinicians in not appropriately diagnosing minority children.

In the face of multiple social and familial risk factors likely to be experienced by Black and Hispanic children compared to White children and even Asian children, culminated with the fact that these children are also more likely to live in substandard neighborhoods with inadequate supply of quality services, one can postulate that Black and Hispanic children with ASD may likely experience less access to services and lower quality services when they get access. When reviewing the early intervention literature, studies show that while Black children are able to access early intervention services and programs, they are also more likely to receive substandard and lower quality programs and services (APA, 2012). In this paper, we put forth a conceptual framework that can be used to guide a research agenda designed to understand why service disparities exist for racial/ethnic minority children with ASD, with the ultimate goal of eliminating said disparities.

First, we describe the components of the Behavioral Model of Health Services Use and past research documenting its effectiveness for examining healthcare utilization. Next, we adapt this model for families of color who have children with ASD and focus on access to educational versus medical or mental health services. Finally, we describe a potential way to move a research agenda forward focused on addressing disparities in access to educational services. We have decided to focus on educational services because this represents the central access point to services for the majority of families who have children with ASD.

2. BEHAVIORAL MODEL OF HEALTH SERVICES USE: A CONCEPTUAL MODEL FOR EXAMINING SERVICE ACCESS AND DISPARITY

Research clearly points to disparities in service access for families of color who have children with ASD (Liptak et al., 2008; Thomas et al., 2007). As stated, these disparities are often exacerbated by issues of income and economic wealth, as children of color in the United States are more likely to live in poverty. In order to improve service access as well as service quality for children of color with ASD, we must better understand the factors that enable and impede access and use for these families. One way to address this issue is through the application of public health models that have been used to examine service utilization in other populations; using this approach would allow the field to forge a research agenda aimed at solving persistent disparities. One of the most well-studied public health models is the Behavioral Model of Health Services Use that Andersen (Andersen, 1968) originally developed. This model has been around for at least 50 years and has been used to examine medical and mental health service access and use in a variety of populations and across illness and disability conditions.

2.1 Overview of the Behavioral Model of Health Services Use

The Behavioral Model of Health Services Use (hereafter referred to as the Behavioral Model) applies a systems perspective to understand why individuals use health services and why there is inequitable access to those services (Andersen, 2008; Phillips, Morrison, Andersen, & Aday, 1998). The model proposes that individual, contextual, and provider level factors all play a role in healthcare utilization. These variables interact with each other and set up bidirectional feedback loops to affect service access and utilization, which ultimately affect health outcomes. The Behavioral Model was first put forth in the 1960's "to assist in defining and measuring multiple dimensions of access to care" (Andersen, 2008, p. 651). It sought to describe the complex relationships between one's predisposition to use services (e.g., a past illness increases the likelihood of future healthcare use), the resources one has that enables him or her to access services, and the person's overall need for care (i.e., How ill are they, or perceive themselves to be?). The model has been expanded over time to include the role of health behavior or lifestyle as well as broader contextual and societal factors that affect healthcare utilization, such as national healthcare policy, changing societal norms and expectations related to being healthy, and geographical distribution of hospitals or other healthcare facilities, to name a few (Andersen, 2008; Andersen & Newman, 2005).

The core of the model has been its focus on what are termed predisposing, enabling and need for care (or illness level) factors (Andersen & Newman, 2005). In earlier versions of the model, the primary focus was on individual determinants of health service utilization, but again, the model has been expanded over time to examine each of these factors at a contextual or societal level as well. Another important expansion of the model was to include provider behaviors that impact service utilization, such as the quality of patient—provider interaction. Andersen (2008) named this category "process of medical care" (p. 652) and it can include other, specific variables such as what tests the provider orders and what counsel or advice is provided to the patient. We now turn to defining each of these factors and some of their related variables. We do not provide details for every variable listed in the original Behavioral Model, both because of space limitations and also to keep the focus on our adapted version of the model (see Fig. 1). For more information on the specific variables included in the original model and/or actual depictions of the model, we refer readers to the following resources: Andersen and Newman, 2005; Andersen, 2008; and Babitsch, Gohl, & von Lengerke, 2012 (full citations are provided in the reference list).

Predisposing factors. Predisposing factors are often ones the individual "comes to the table with" and thus are more difficult to change, but nonetheless serve as important predictors of healthcare utilization. In essence, these are variables that predispose one to seek out services and often exist prior to actual illness onset (Andersen & Newman, 2005). In the Behavioral Model, there are three broad categories of variables under the predisposing factor— demographic, social structure and health beliefs. The demographic and social structure categories are often discussed as societal or individual determinants of health in the broader public health field (Andersen & Newman, 2005; Babitsch et al., 2012). Andersen and Newman include four variables in the demographic category: age, sex, marital status and past illness. The basic proposition is that these demographic factors predispose individuals to seek out (or not) healthcare services. For instance, as individuals age, they are more likely to experience health-related complications, and therefore, seek out healthcare services. There is sometimes an interaction between age and sex with some research indicating that younger men are less likely to visit a doctor and women, overall, being more likely to utilize healthcare services (Babitsch et al., 2012). For young men, feelings of invincibility combined with their perceptions of masculinity can contribute to their decreased likelihood of seeking medical attention (Jeffries & Grogan, 2012). While there can be cultural and geographic differences that affect how well marital status predicts healthcare utilization, in general, it has been found that those who are married are more likely to routinely use healthcare. Lastly, past illness predicts healthcare utilization because those who have been ill, in particular if they experience some chronic illness or ongoing medical condition, will be more prone to need healthcare in the future.

The social structure variables represent one's social status or positioning in society, which also affects the likelihood an individual will seek out services. In a socially stratified society, issues of race and class certainly affect an individual's ability and propensity to seek and secure healthcare services. In the original model, there are a total of six variables listed under this category (i.e., education, race/ethnicity, occupation, family size, religion, and residential mobility). We simply highlight a few relevant variables here to provide context for how social structure variables can impact healthcare access and utilization. Race/ethnicity has consistently been identified as a determining factor in healthcare seeking behavior (Andersen et al., 2002; Babitsch et al., 2012; Dhingra, Zack, Strine, Pearson, & Balluz, 2010), with racial/ethnic minorities, in particular those who experience disenfranchisement based on their racial status being less likely to access services. Further, in the U.S., one's occupation affects the availability and cost of private health insurance, and thus the person's ability to access affordable healthcare. While it may seem odd to include religion in this category, in US society, some religions are more socially accepted than others. In fact, some religious communities are at odds with societal norms because they discourage their parishioners from using some forms of traditional medicines and therapies (e.g., Jehovah's Witnesses' refusals of blood transfusions; Viele & Weiskopf, 1994). Finally, both demographic and social structure variables often impact one's health beliefs and attitudes (Andersen & Newman, 2005); thus, the final category included under the predisposing factor was health beliefs, which includes the specific variables of one's values concerning health and illness, attitudes toward health services, and knowledge of one's disease. Health beliefs are relevant because they can impact healthcare utilization. For example, if a person believes that homeopathic or alternative therapies are a better remedy for certain conditions or illnesses, then they are less likely to use traditional healthcare services. In the updated model that considers context, the same three broad categories of variables are included but also are considered at the aggregate or population level. For instance, instead of considering just the individual's race, the racial composition of one's community or neighborhood could be examined as a predisposing factor. Racially segregated neighborhoods with high concentrations of racial/ethnic minority populations are more likely to have access to substandard hospitals and schools (Gaskin, Zare, Halder & LaVeis, 2016; Williams & Jackson, 2005); thus, decreasing the quality of services provided and the likelihood of repeatedly accessing those services.

Enabling factors. Enabling factors are those that permit the individual to secure needed services. These factors are also most likely to contribute to inequitable access to services. In the Behavioral Model, enabling factors are considered at both the family/individual and community level. Family level variables include ones that are now considered pretty standard in determining healthcare utilization, such as household income, health insurance coverage and whether one has a regular source of healthcare and routine access to that care (Andersen & Newman, 2008). Basic access to health insurance has been found to be a predictor of mental health treatment as well (Dhingra et al., 2010). Community level variables include the number of healthcare facilities and personnel relative to the size of community that needs to be served, the price of healthcare, and geographic variables, including the region of the country where one resides. Other researchers have included such variables as access to transportation in order to reach a healthcare facility, wait time to receive care, and organizational barriers that could include such issues as the doctor's office hours or the type of providers available at a given facility (Babitsch et al., 2012).

Need for care factors. In Andersen and Newman (2005), they differentiate two variables that comprise the need for care factor. Those variables are *perceived* and *evaluated* need for healthcare. Perceived need refers to the individual's perception of how healthy or ill they are, in essence, to what extent do they perceive themselves to need medical care. The variables under perceived need include the number of disability or sick days an individual has taken, the symptoms the individual has experienced over a period of time, prior diagnoses received, and the person's overall health or general state of well-being. Evaluated need refers to independent, clinical verification of the individual's symptoms, conditions or diagnoses. Of course, conflicts between perceived and evaluated need can arise, and how those conflicts are resolved also can impact healthcare utilization. For example, if a child is evaluated for and diagnosed with ASD; however, the parents don't agree with the diagnosis, then that will affect their course of action regarding treatment. At the contextual level, the need for care factor includes conditions related to environmental health and safety (e.g., How crime-ridden is the community; How polluted is the air or water?) and population level health indices of a given community (e.g., What is the overall level of disability, mortality and morbidity?).

Outcomes. The outcomes included in the Behavioral Model align with its need for care factor in that both focus on the notion of perceived versus evaluated. With the need for care factor, these variables related to the person's subjective opinion of his/her illness and how those perceptions did (or did not) align with the clinical evaluations of trained professionals. With outcomes, the focus is on whether the person now perceives themselves to be healthy or recovered, and again, if those perceptions correspond with objective tests. The final variable included under outcomes is consumer satisfaction, as clients or patients are unlikely to continue to use services if they are unhappy with the results. As such, the model depicts a bidirectionality between both the contextual and individual characteristics and outcomes, which as Andersen stated, "introduces the dynamic and recursive nature of a health services use model that includes health status outcomes (Andersen, 2008, p. 652).

2.2 Relevant Research on the Behavioral Model

Babitsch et al. (2012) conducted a systematic review of studies where the Behavioral Model had been used as the framework for examining healthcare utilization. Their review included 16 studies published in English or German between 1998 and 2011. Here, we highlight some relevant findings from their systematic review (please see the original article for more extensive detail) that could be applicable to families of color who have children with ASD. First, it has been found that in the US, racial/ethnic minority status does impact healthcare utilization, with Black non-Hispanics, Hispanics, Asians and other racial/ethnic groups being less likely to receive treatment than their White, non-Hispanic counterparts (Andersen et al., 2002; Blackwell, Martinez, Gentleman, Sanmartin, & Berthelot, 2009; Dhingra et al., 2010). Second, lower education levels and income status are associated with less frequent use of healthcare services (Andersen et al., 2002; Blackwell et al., 2009), albeit the relationship with income is not always straightforward (Dhingra et al., 2010), because income is often related to other variables like race/ethnicity, as racial minorities tend to have lower incomes and wealth than their White counterparts. Still, one study found that African-American men from the lowest education group, in particular, were less likely to be regularly seen by a healthcare professional (Hammond, Matthews, Gorbie-Smith, 2010). Finally, another relevant finding is that health beliefs or cultural norms can play a role in the decision to seek treatment (Insaf, Jurkowski, & Alomar, 2010). As previously stated, we know that in the US there is an unfortunate intersection between race and class; and thus, for families of color who have a child with a disability, issues of race, education, income and cultural beliefs are also likely to affect their ability to access high quality services as well as their decision-making processes about which services to utilize.

As first stated in the introduction to this paper, children of color in the US are more likely to receive harsher disciplinary consequences in school settings and there is a long-standing history of Black boys, in particular, being tracked into segregated, special education services (Harry & Anderson, 1994). Yet, we often fail to consider how being a multiple minority, in this instance being a racial/ethnic minority and having a disability, intersect to affect outcomes. Further, we often primarily focus our efforts on the role of poverty in explaining achievement gaps and related educational disparities (O'Connor & Fernandez, 2006), but this fails to consider other structural forces, for example, systematic racism that are also likely to be contributing factors. Erevelles and Minear (2010) encourage us to consider the intersection among these "multiply minoritizing identities" (p. 127), such as race, class, and disability, as well as the ways that larger social institutions (e.g., the educational system) can contribute to and promulgate oppression and disparities. In our proposed model (described below), we attempt to consider the child in his or her totality, i.e., both as a child of color and a child with a disability.

2.3 Summary

The Behavioral Model of Health Services Use is a widely-used and empirically supported framework for examining healthcare utilization. It has been used to identify individual, societal and contextual determinants that contribute to healthcare seeking and use behaviors in a variety of populations and across healthcare conditions. In general, the way equitable, or rather inequitable, service access is determined using the Behavioral Model is through quantitative data analysis, that is, inequitable access to services occurs if most of the variance in healthcare utilization is explained by *social structure, health beliefs and enabling variables* rather than need for care factors or the specific demographic variables included in the model, such as age or past illness. This model has applicability to families of color who have children with ASD because these families likely face similar demographic and structural forces that would affect their ability to access high quality services.

2.4 Model of School-Based Service Access for Children of Color With ASD

We have chosen to adapt the Behavioral Model of Health Services Use to apply it to families of color who have children with ASD in order to examine their ability to access school-based services. We present this model to guide services research, and potentially practice, in the field. We know that disparities in service access exist for economically disadvantaged and racial/ethnic minority families who have children with ASD; thus so far, we have been able to detect or identify those disparities. Based on Kilbourne and colleagues' (Kilbourne, Switzer, Hyman, Crowley-Matoka, & Fine, 2006) work related to health disparities research, the next stage of research after detection is to *understand why* disparities exist. This adapted framework should allow us to begin to answer that question (see Fig. 1).

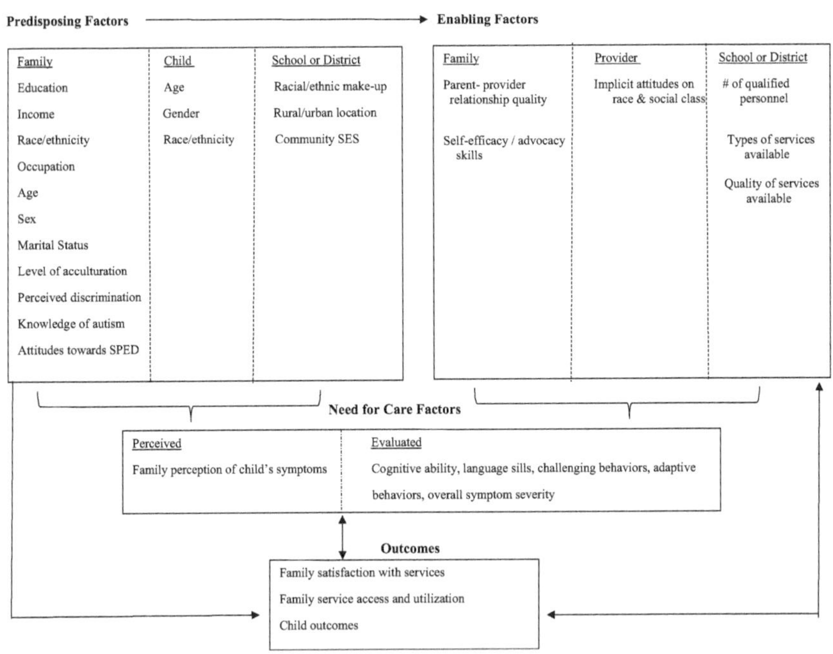

Figure 1 Adapted model of school-based service access for children of color with ASD

Predisposing factors. In our adapted model, we have chosen to organize the predisposing factors by *family/parent characteristics, child characteristics* and *school characteristics*, because we argue that all of these predisposing factors interact to affect parents' likelihood of accessing school-based services for their child with ASD. For *family/parent characteristics*, we have maintained many of the demographic and social structure variables that were included in the original model. While we know less in ASD research about how issues of parent age, sex and marital status affect service access, these are certainly relevant demographic variables in US society and, in general, predict service utilization (Babitsch et al., 2012). In addition, parental age and sex are variables associated with ASD diagnoses in that advanced paternal and maternal age have been associated with increased odds of having a child with the disorder (Lee & McGrath, 2015), and thus a need to seek out services. Further, we know from research on the original Behavioral Model that the social structure variables of education, income, race/ethnicity and occupation all interact to affect healthcare utilization (Babitsch et al., 2012). It should be noted that in the original model income is included as an enabling factor and we have moved it to the predisposing category. We have done so because families do not have to pay for public school-based, special education services; thus, income should not directly enable (or disable) a parent from accessing services. However, in ASD, there appears to be a complex interaction between such parent variables as race and income status and parent perception of the impact of their children's diagnosis. A longitudinal study of 30 Black families of children with ASD at 9 and 14 years of age found that Black mothers reported less of a negative impact from rearing a child with ASD than White mothers (Bishop, Richler, Cain, & Lord, 2007), with low-income Black mothers reporting the least impact (Carr & Lord, 2013). If low-income parents perceive less of an impact of the child's ASD diagnosis on the family, then this may decrease their motivation to seek services. Relatedly, in a study on self-perception of social status, White families of children with ASD self-reported a higher social status, in particular when compared to Latino families (Manning, Wainwright, & Bennett, 2011). Having a higher social status affects the types of resources available to the family to support (or educate) the parent about ASD as well as the parent's ability to procure effective services for the child. Parents' race/ethnicity and socioeconomic status (i.e. income and education level) then become relevant variables to consider in families' service access for their children with ASD.

Importantly, we have added some variables to our family/parent characteristic composite, including level of acculturation, perceived discrimination, knowledge of ASD and child development, and attitudes towards special education. Level of acculturation or social capital, in general, has been found to be a factor that affects the advocacy and engagement of minority families with the special education system (Boyd & Correa, 2005; Harry, Allen, & McLaughlin, 1995). We know less about the direct effect of discrimination on families of color who have children with ASD. Still research from other disciplines indicates that perceived discrimination is related to parenting behaviors (Dotterer & Lowe, 2015), and therefore, likely to affect parents' propensity to engage with the school system, perhaps to a greater extent since school providers are often of a different race. Parents' knowledge of ASD and child development, such as their understanding about the causes of symptoms (e.g. Are behavior problems related to characteristics associated with ASD or the child being "spoiled"?) and important developmental milestones, also could influence the services they perceive their child to need (Mandell & Novak, 2005). Finally, parents' perceptions and attitudes about the effectiveness of school-based, special education services are likely to have an impact on their desire to seek out and advocate for those services.

The *child characteristics* included in the model are age, race and gender. We included these variables because they are associated with a child with ASD receiving a later diagnosis, and later diagnosis translates to delayed access to services. The average age of diagnosis is still around four years of age and racial/ethnic minority children (Liptak et al., 2008; Kogan et al., 2009) and girls (Dworzynski, Ronald, Bolton, & Happe 2012) are still at risk for being diagnosed at later ages or misdiagnosed. The included *school characteristics* are analogous to the contextual variables included in the original model, but here we consider more aggregate level variables at the school or school district level. Schools with higher concentrations of racial/ethnic minority children and schools located in rural or inner city, urban areas are more likely to be low-resourced schools and have fewer qualified personnel (Reardon, 2016). Finally, we know that school funding in the US is related to the zip code and socioeconomic status of the neighborhood in which its located, which impacts the availability and quality of services.

Enabling factors. For enabling factors, we again take a multiple levels of influence approach to understand what impacts the parent's ability to secure needed school-based services. We also propose that some parent and provider variables may be more amenable to change via intervention, and these "mutable factors" will act as more proximal contributors to family access to services, and ultimately children's improved outcomes. The mutable parent factors identified as enablers of access to services include parent self-efficacy/advocacy and quality of the parent-provider relationship. Self-efficacy is thought to play a mediating role between thought and action (Bandura, 1989). For example, parents of color may be more persistent in accessing services for their child if they believe they will be successful. Low self-efficacy may lead parents to advocate less for appropriate services, especially if they encounter difficulties. However, we know it is possible through intervention to teach parents effective advocacy strategies (Burke, Goldman, Hart, & Hodapp, 2016) for interacting with school system personnel. Further, positive parent-school provider relationships are less common for low-income and racial minority families (Entwisle & Alexander, 1988; Hughes & Oi-man, 2007). As a result, we must understand how these relationships impact service access and children's outcomes. Thus, it is important to examine the role of factors such as self-efficacy and provider-parent relationships to better understand the engagement and sustained involvement of racial/ethnic minority parents in advocating for services for their children with ASD.

The provider factors included as enablers in our model are largely based on the work of Cooper et al. (2012). Through a line of research on minority health disparities, she has found that Black patients' perceptions of racism or discrimination from their physicians as well as the physicians' implicit attitudes on race and class contribute to less patient-centered care (Boulware, Cooper, Ratner, LaVeist, & Rowe, 2003; Cooper et al., 2012; Johnson, Roter, Powe, & Cooper, 2004). This is important because better patient-centered care has been linked to improved patients' perceptions of their providers (Cooper et al., 2009, 2011, 2012) and health outcomes for minorities (Kaplan, Greenfield, & Ware, 1989; Little et al., 2001; Stewart, 1995). Racial/ethnic minority families who have children with ASD are dependent upon school system providers to help inform decisions about appropriate care and services. Thus, it becomes important to understand the impact of school providers' implicit biases on minority families' ability to access services and improve children's outcomes. In ASD, we know so little about how issues of cultural diversity affect family or child outcomes, or the ways in which diversity facilitate or inhibit the ability of families to access appropriate services for their children. Yet, such information could be critical for the development of culturally-tailored interventions and play a pivotal role in improving access to services and outcomes for children of color with ASD. It is our belief that service providers are not purposefully attempting to discriminate against families of color who have children with ASD. However, research suggests that such factors as the family's cultural capital/social concordance with providers, i.e. the degree to which the parent and provider are of similar education level, income and race, does have an impact on provider-client relationships (Thornton, Rowe, Roter & Cooper, 2011). Poor quality relationships with providers may lead parents to have indifferent or even adversarial interactions with providers, and in turn, could lead providers to develop implicit (or subconscious) negative stereotypes about certain families. We know less about the role of these attitudinal variables on minority families' ability to access school-based services for their child with ASD. Importantly, research has found that implicit attitudes can be changed through cognitive processes (e.g. visual imagery, role-playing) that provide exposure to positive exemplars of a devalued group (Dasgupta & Greenwald, 2001).

When discussing implicit attitudes, there is a question of how one measures subconscious biases; yet, objective tests of implicit bias do exist. One such tool is the Implicit Associations Test (IAT), which can be used to measure a variety of forms of implicit bias including level of subconscious bias related to race (IAT-R) and social class (IAT-S) (Greenwald, McGhee, & Schwartz, 1998). The IAT is administered via computer and assesses implicit attitudes by measuring the response latency and errors associated with individuals sorting words from four concepts into only two categories (e.g. Black vs. White). The IAT has been used in minority health disparities research to assess the implicit racial attitudes of physicians. Cooper et al. (2012) found that among Black patients, physicians' implicit racial biases were associated with more verbal dominance by the physician during interactions, less positive affect exhibited by the patient and poorer ratings of interpersonal care. Prior data on the IAT also indicate it is sensitive to the attitudes of teachers. Elementary and secondary teachers ($n = 2000$) scored a mean of 0.34 on the IAT-R and the normative mean for the measure is 0.30 (personal communication, Project Implicit, 2012), indicating that teachers may have somewhat higher levels of implicit bias than found in the general population. Finally, we have included the school contextual variables of the number of qualified personnel and the types and quality of services available (e.g., Are inclusive classrooms even an option?) in a given school or district to serve children with ASD. For example, Irvin and colleagues (Irvin, McBee, Boyd, Hume, & Odom, 2012) found that Hispanic children with ASD were less likely to receive school-based speech and language or occupational therapy services when compared to White children; the authors postulated that this may be due to the lack of trained bilingual therapists to serve the specific needs of these students. In summary, we suggest that family, provider and school-level variables all interact to affect the ability of parents of color to secure needed services for their child with ASD.

Need for care factors. We have maintained Andersen's distinction between evaluated and perceived need because parent perceptions of their child's symptoms could impact their service seeking behavior. Under evaluated need, we include the behaviors and skills that affect the functioning level of a child with ASD, i.e., cognitive ability, language skills, challenging behavior, adaptive behavior, and overall symptom severity. All of these domains can be evaluated with objective tests by expert clinicians. We include perceived need because research has pointed to some discrepancy over the relationship between race/ethnicity and parent perception of children's symptoms. Blacher et al. (2014) found that Latina mothers under-reported their child's ASD symptoms in comparison to White mothers, even though Latino children had higher scores on observed measures of autism symptomatology. In contrast, Liptak et al. (2008) found that ethnically and socioeconomically diverse parents were more likely to over-report their child's ASD symptoms. Certainly, parents' *perceptions* of the child's behaviors and symptoms can influence their actions, and if they perceive their child to be less symptomatic then the parent may choose to not access school-based services.

Outcomes. We focused on three primary outcomes in our adapted model: family satisfaction with services, family service access and utilization, and child outcomes. The family satisfaction with services variable is in direct alignment with the original Behavioral Model (Andersen, 2008). One of the outcomes of the family's ability to more easily access and use school-based services should be increased satisfaction with the educational system and school providers. We stray from the Behavioral Model in our purposeful inclusion of service access and utilization as an actual outcome variable in our model. We have done so because the focus is not just on the identification of barriers to service access, but also on the enabling, or rather mutable, factors that can be changed to ultimately improve a parent's ability to access and use effective services for their children. Further, for child outcomes, there is not a distinction between evaluated and perceived outcomes in our model. We view this as a bit of false separation when it relates to outcomes, as our belief is that if parents and providers have a better relationship, parents have the skills and knowledge to advocate for their child, providers have less implicit bias related to some families, and the services are available at a given school, then these variables should interact to increase agreement between parents and providers about children's improvement. For clarification, when we refer to child outcomes those include the broad range of educational, developmental and behavioral outcomes one would expect improved when a child receives school-based services. Our adapted model is also slightly different in how we view bidirectionality between some of the factors. Unlike the Behavioral Model, we did not include bidirectional arrows between the predisposing factors and outcomes. We did this because the predisposing factors included in our model largely centered on demographic and structural variables and left out the health belief variables; thus, the majority of these variables are not amenable to change (e.g., one's race/ethnicity), and even if changed, those changes are not as likely to have resulted from improved outcomes. For example, a person may gain more formal education, but it is doubtful that she or he did that because of increased satisfaction with the child's educational services. However, the bidirectionality between the enabling and need for care factors and outcomes are maintained, as in the original model.

2.5 Summary

Our adapted Model of School-Based Service Access for Children of Color with ASD has many parallels to the Behavioral Model with its focus on predisposing, enabling and need for care factors, and how those factors interact to affect family and child outcomes. Most of the modifications to our model are related to examining the educational versus health care system in the United States. Further, our model is focused on the ability of racially/ethnically diverse families to access services, and thus includes some variables that may affect these families more, such as, perceived discrimination, level of acculturation, and the implicit biases of school providers. Finally, it must be noted that our model has not been empirically validated; therefore, we now turn to proposing a future research agenda focused on understanding why disparities in service access exist for minority families of children with ASD, with the ultimate goal of eliminating those disparities.

3. CHARTING THE PATH FORWARD: A RESEARCH AGENDA FOCUSED ON UNDERSTANDING DISPARITIES IN EDUCATIONAL SERVICES ACCESS IN ASD

First, it must be acknowledged that as with the original Behavioral Model, the adapted model could be studied using observational or experimental study designs or statistical analyses that allow one to examine the variance explained by the various factors. We also assert that inequitable access is likely best determined if service access and utilization are best explained by enabling factors rather than need for care factors. Yet, it is our belief that there are some important considerations when examining school service access for children of color with ASD. We touch on three important concepts (i.e., social concordance, service negotiation and implicit bias) and also make recommendations for how to measure them in order to lay out a research agenda. We have previously described social concordance and implicit bias but elaborate on them here because of their likely importance to understanding school service disparities for families of color with ASD.

3.1 Social Concordance

Social concordance has been used to examine the role of race and other demographic variables on patient—physician interaction (Thornton, Powe, Roter, & Cooper, 2011). To measure it, social concordance is often examined as a composite score based on the degree to which there is a match (or degree of similarity) on basic demographic variables between the patient (for school services research, the parent) and physician (for school services research, the primary teacher). Some of the traditional social concordance demographic variables included in studies are age, race/ethnicity, gender and education level.

Social concordance is important to consider in educational research because multiple studies note a cultural mismatch (e.g., communicative style; Gumperz & Cook-Gumperz, 1981, pp. 430—445) between teachers and parents, which can have implications for how teachers view their children (Hughes, Gleason, & Zhang, 2005). In the public health field, it has been found that dissimilarity between providers and clients on such factors as race/ethnicity can lead to more client dissatisfaction with services (Cooper-Patrick et al., 1999; Thornton et al., 2011). Based on workforce statistics (U.S. Department of Education, National Center for Education Statistics, 2013), over 84% of public school teachers are White; thus, there is a high degree of racial *dis*cordance with racially/ethnically diverse families. We do expect gender concordance between the parent and teacher because mothers are often primary caretakers of children, and approximately 75% of the teaching workforce is female. Another demographic variable that may be important to consider when examining social concordance between parents and providers is primary language spoken. There is a growing need for bilingual educators and communication barriers between parents and providers likely impact service access.

3.2 Service Negotiation

While evidence exists about the importance of involving the perspectives of families in the service negotiation process, research often highlights the limited engagement of low-income and ethnic minority families (Boethel, 2003; Hill et al., 2004; Wong & Hughes, 2006). Various reasons exist for these families' limited engagement compared to White and higher incomes families, ranging from their availability to meet because of atypical work schedules, lack of transportation and child care; and more importantly, for families with children with disabilities not feeling valued and included in the process (Jo Landmark, Zhang, & Montoya, 2007; Lamb-Parker et al., 2001). We know that ethnic minority children with ASD and children from lower income households are at risk for poorer outcomes in comparison to their White and higher income counterparts, including a more severe symptom presentation (e.g., more severe language & cognitive delays) (Centers for Disease Control and Prevention, 2014; Cuccaro et al., 2007; Fountain et al., 2012). One posited rationale for poor outcomes for ethnic minority and low-income children is the receipt of lower quality or fewer services. As research emerges about how and when to detect ASD, there is a need to better understand how to ensure that all children with ASD, especially ethnic minority children and those from low-income households, access high quality services after detection. The negotiation process for determining services for children in the United States, which predominantly occurs during the legally-mandated, school-based Individualized Education Plan (IEP) meetings, is instrumental for children to receive appropriate and high-quality services (Gartin & Murdick, 2005). Further, the inclusion of families during service negotiation is instrumental in ensuring that the goals, expectations, and assessments are appropriate and meet the needs of the child and support their improvement (Byington & Whitby, 2011; Ruppar & Gaffney, 2011). One of the question then becomes — How does one study the service negotiation process?

Assessing the quality of the service negotiation process. Family centeredness is a core component of determining whether the service negotiation process is of high quality. However, there is limited knowledge about the actual discourse related to decision-making that occurs during the service negotiation process despite the importance of IEP meetings in the lives of children with disabilities and their families (Ruppar & Gaffney, 2011). Some research has evaluated the quality of IEP goals and outcomes (Lynch & Beare, 1990; Ruble, McGrew, Dalrymple, & Jung, 2010), but very little research has assessed the quality of the negotiation process, while making an effort to include the parents' perspectives (Childre & Chambers, 2005). One existing tool to examine the IEP meeting – IEP Observation Record (Davis, 1983) – while covering multiple areas, such as child educational placement and legal rights, is limited in its examination of family-centered processes. There are no known research-based, objective tools to examine the quality of the service negotiation process. This has subsequently led to the sole use of parent or teacher reports, and in some instances the produced IEPs, as a way to ascertain the quality of the negotiation process. Multiple studies from various areas, including public health, medicine, and social science note that while parent and teacher information are valuable and provide unique information, they are at best moderately correlated (Cai, Kaiser, & Hancock, 2004; Greenfield, Iruka, & Munis, 2004) and often contain biases which are likely impacted by the relationship as well as individual's characteristics (e.g., race/ethnicity, social class) (Iruka, Winn, Kingsley, & Orthodoxou, 2011). Finally, the service negation process, and thus the quality of the IEP, is likely influenced by the relationship the parents and teachers have with each other prior to this formal meeting (IEP meetings most often occur later in the school year). Unfortunately, as noted, positive parent-teacher relationships are less common for low-income and racial minority families (Hughes & Oi-man, 2007). Thus, we propose the adoption of a system has been used within the conduct of physician–patient interactions – the Roter Interaction Analysis System (RIAS; Roter & Hall, 1992).

Use of the RIAS to assess service negotiation quality. Measuring the quality of the parent-teacher/educational team interaction during the IEP negotiation process is one way to understand whether families of color with children with ASD can access high quality services; however, no valid means of objectively capturing this process currently exist. The RIAS has been used extensively to examine patient-doctor interactions during clinic visits to determine whether verbal and nonverbal communication was patient-centered and if patients were satisfied with their visit. The RIAS is based on social exchange theory focused on interpersonal influence, problem solving and reciprocity; it captures the extent to which the communication between patients (parents for school-based research) and physicians (teachers and educational teams for school-based research) is tasked-focused and includes social-emotional content. The system assigns utterance codes to 1 of 37 mutually exclusive categories of communication in the areas of data gathering (e.g., open- and close-ended questions), education and counseling, relationship-building (e.g., empathy, concern, criticism), and partnership building (seeking opinion and checking for understanding). In addition to the utterances, coders rate the affect or emotional contexts of the speakers in the areas of dominance, assertiveness, friendliness, warmth, attentiveness, and respectfulness. The RIAS has demonstrated reliability and predictive validity in studies of patient—physician communication with reported inter-coder reliability coefficients averaging 0.85 and is predictive of physician and patient satisfaction (Roter & Larson, 2001). The RIAS has been used extensively in the medical field to improve practitioners' patient-centeredness (e.g., Cavaco & Roter, 2010; Cooper et al., 2011). While used in a medical setting, it still has been noted to be practical and time efficient, functional, flexible, and adaptive to medical situations (e.g., well-baby care, end of life discussions). Considering some of the similarities between patient-doctor and parent-teacher interactions, where parents (and patients) are seeking information and advocating for services in a collaborative fashion with their child's teacher (and doctors), we expect that the RIAS would be able to capture the extent to which the service negotiation process during IEP meetings is accessible and empathetic to parents with limited professional jargon and allows for parents to ask questions and share their values, goals, and expectations for their child. Finally, the RIAS has been used within the context of family conferences such as to examine difficult conversations between NICU clinicians and parents (Boss, Donohue, Larson, Arnold, & Roter, 2016); thus, it likely can be applied to IEP team meetings, with the meeting being audiotaped and later coded using the RIAS coding system. The coding system generates quite a bit of output including type of talk that providers and patients engage in (e.g., gives medical information, gives lifestyle information, makes personal remarks, makes critical remarks, asks opinion, expresses concern); percentage of time different individuals talked; and based, in part, on the coding of provider(s) versus patient talk, a "patient-centeredness" score can be derived. A noted limitation of using RIAS within the context of IEP meetings is that school providers and/or parents may be resistant to those meetings being audiotaped given potential legal ramifications as well as the sensitive nature of topics that may be discussed.

3.3 Implicit Bias

Implicit bias is a concept that has been well-studied in social psychology (Greenwald & Banaji, 1995), but we are only beginning to examine its impact within educational contexts. Implicit bias refers to mental associations linking social groups to stereotypic attributes. These associations form the basis for stereotypic thoughts and feelings that come to mind involuntarily, i.e., independent of whether a person consciously believes or rejects those thoughts and feelings. Unlike explicit bias, in which thoughts and feelings are consciously considered and voluntarily reported using questionnaires, implicit bias is often measured using objective behavioral tests, such as the aforementioned IAT (https://implicit.harvard.edu/implicit/). Studies suggest that implicit bias is much more prevalent than explicit bias, either because respondents consciously reject such biases or because they wish to present themselves as an unbiased person on explicit measures (Nosek, Banaji, & Greenwald, 2002). Implicit bias predicts a range of intergroup behaviors, even after controlling for explicit bias. For example, individuals higher in implicit race bias tend to be less friendly in interactions with a Black conversation partner (Dovidio, Kawakami, & Gaertner, 2002). Further, implicit bias is associated with less positive physician–patient interactions (Penner et al., 2010); with biased criminal sentencing among jurors (Blair, Judd, & Fallman, 2004) and judges (Rachlinski, Johnson, Wistrich, & Guthrie, 2009); and with biased personnel decisions in hiring (Ziegert & Hanges, 2005). Together, the findings indicate that implicit bias is a risk factor for discriminatory treatment even among individuals who consciously reject such bias. It is important to note that education level is not associated with implicit bias, although it is associated with explicit bias. More educated individuals have similar implicit biases to those with less education, but they are less likely to report those attitudes explicitly (Kuppens & Spears, 2014). Thus, implicit bias may be an important pathway by which racial/ethnic and class disparities are maintained despite gradual reductions in explicit prejudice.

Association between implicit bias and child outcomes. Relatively few studies have examined the impact of implicit bias on educational outcomes (Staats & Patton, 2013), and we are not aware of any research focused on children of color with ASD. Based on experimental studies, it has been demonstrated that teachers prescribe harsher disciplinary consequences to typically developing children *perceived* as Black versus White for committing the same infraction (La Vonne, McCray, Webb-Johnson, & Bridgest, 2003; Okonofua & Eberhardt, 2015). For example, researchers at Stanford University recruited racially diverse K-12 teachers ($n = 57$) to view the fictitious school discipline records of students with stereotypically Black or White names (Okonofua & Eberhardt, 2015). These fictitious records indicated that students had committed the same two infractions; however, teachers who reviewed the records of students with "Black" names tended to recommend harsher disciplinary consequences for a second infraction and describe this second infraction as being indicative of a behavioral pattern. Of note, the relationship between student race and recommended disciplinary consequence was partially mediated by teachers' implicit judgments of Black students as "troublemakers." Naturalistic studies also have confirmed the impact of implicit bias on educational outcomes. A study conducted in the Netherlands comparing elementary-aged, native Dutch students to racial/ethnic minority students (total n = 434) found that teachers held more negative implicit attitudes toward minority students, and in those classrooms where this occurred, there were larger achievement gaps on standardized tests (Van den Bergh, Denessen, Hornstra, Voeten, & Holland, 2010). Further, in this study, teachers' implicit biases but not explicit prejudicial attitudes were associated with student outcomes, indicating that explicit measures are likely more prone to social desirability effects. Finally, these researchers found that teacher expectations mediated the relationship between implicit biases and child outcomes. Thus, implicit biases may not only impact providers' interactions with racially and ethnically diverse parents, as described in the adapted conceptual model, but also has the potential to directly impact the outcomes of children of color with ASD.

3.4 Charting a Research Agenda

We have described three concepts that may be important to consider when embarking on a research agenda related to understanding why service access disparities exist for children of color with ASD. It is also important to consider the types of studies that are still needed to address some of these pressing research questions and issues. First, there is a dearth of longitudinal studies in the field focused on families of color who have children with ASD. Longitudinal research is needed to help us understand how service access for children with ASD changes over time in relation to changes in child symptoms (or other variables), and what are the important mediating variables that may account for any changes in the relationship between service access and children's outcomes (e.g., decreases in providers' implicit biases over time).

Further, there is a need to think differently about intervention research because to ultimately impact service access we have to intervene at the level of the school system as well as provider and parent. These sort of multi-level interventions are more prevalent within the context of public health but have not been as readily applied within educational research. One example within educational research that could be relevant is the work being done to

Bridge the Word Gap for children in poverty (Greenwood et al., 2017) who are at-risk for poorer outcomes because they hear fewer words from their parents during critical periods of early childhood development. This group has proposed community-level interventions that could involve various sectors and entities, for example education and business, and propose to examine the impact of the intervention at multiple levels in order to understand impact and scale-up.

4. CONCLUSION

The Behavioral Model has provided a foundation to better understand inequity in access for health-related services. Using a similar approach, we present a conceptual model, adapted from the early works of Andersen, in order to examine the ability of families of color with children with ASD to access school-based services. Issues regarding how these families' access school-based services for young children with ASD have been previously examined, but with limited attempt to understand why such inequities have disproportionately impacted families of color. To the best of our knowledge, this is the first attempt to guide future research and practice in the field by providing a conceptual model in order to examine factors that enable or impede school-related access for ethnic minorities with the ultimate goal of eliminating these disparities.

Notably, an attempt has been made to account for such factors as acculturation, perceived discrimination, and implicit bias when examining access to school-based services. We believe these factors are relevant for accessing school-based services and may explain some of the reported disparities for children of color when compared to their White, more affluent peers. Further, this model represents an attempt to increase empirical data on families of color and educational disparities by presenting a framework that can now be validated in future studies, and by suggesting the types of study designs that are needed, such as more longitudinal studies on racial/ethnic minority families. We do recognize there are limitations associated with our proposed model. For instance, this model is focused on school-based services; however, these families often interact with multiple service systems and agencies, such as Medicaid. It is often the disjointedness and lack of coordination between different services systems that contribute to parents' frustrations and gaps in service access (Boyd, Odom, Humphreys, & Sam, 2010). Further, our model is likely most applicable to preschool and elementary-aged children with ASD; yet, we know that as children with ASD age the complexity and number of services families may need to access grow and change over time. As families have to become familiar with vocational rehabilitation services to help their child find appropriate employment supports (Kochhar-Bryant & Izzo, 2006), or more familiar with healthcare as their child transitions from the pediatric to the adult healthcare system (Cooley & Sagerman, 2011).

Still, we posit that such a model is needed to guide research in the field and to guide practice back towards more family-centered, school-based care. Dunst and Trivette (1996) define family-centeredness as "a particular set of beliefs, principles, values, and practices for supporting and strengthening family capacity to enhance and promote child development and learning." School systems are already familiar with the concepts of child and family-centered approaches regulated under Part C of the Individuals with Disabilities Education Act (IDEA, 2004); however, we often move away from this model of care as children transition from Part C (early intervention focused; birth - 3) to Part B (school-based focused; 3–21) services. Importantly, family-centered practices are associated with positive child and family outcomes, including higher parent self-efficacy and program satisfaction (Byington & Whitby, 2011; Dunst, Trivette, & Hamby, 2007). Thus, revisiting this approach and applying it to children and families of color is appropriate. Family centeredness should be used to help address variables that promote equitable access to school-related services. Such application of a family-centered approach may ultimately improve parent-provider relationships and positively impact long-term outcomes for children with ASD.

REFERENCES

American Psychological Association, Presidential Task Force on Educational Disparities. (2012). *Ethnic and racial disparities in education: Psychology's contributions to understanding and reducing disparities*. Retrieved from: http://www.apa.org/ed/resources/racial-disparities.aspx.

Andersen, R. (1968). *A behavioral model of families' use of health services. A behavioral model of families' use of health services*. Chicago, IL: Center for Health Administration Studies, University of Chicago. Research Series No. 25.

Andersen, R. (2008). National health surveys and the behavioral model of health service use. *Medical Care, 46*(7), 647–653.

Andersen, R., Yu, H., Wyn, R., Davidson, P. L., Brown, E. R., & Teleki, S. (2002). Access to medical care for low-income persons: How do communities make a difference? *Medical Care Research and Review: MCRR, 59*(4), 384–411.

Andersen, R., & Newman, J. F. (2005). Societal and individual determinants of medical care utilization in the United States. *The Milbank Quarterly, 83*(4), 1–28.

Aud, S., Fox, M. A., & KewalRamani, A. (2010). Status and Trends in the Education of Racial and Ethnic Groups. NCES 2010-015. *National Center for Education Statistics*.

Babitsch, B., Gohl, D., & von Lengerke, T. (2012). Re-revisiting Andersen's behavioral model of health service use: A systematic review of studies from 1998–2011. *Psycho-Social-Medicine, 9*.

Bandura, A. (1989). Regulation of cognitive processes through perceived self-efficacy. *Developmental Psychology, 25*(5), 729.

Bishop, S. L., Richler, J., Cain, A. C., & Lord, C. (2007). Predictors of perceived negative impact in mothers of children with autism spectrum disorder. *American Journal on Mental Retardation, 112*(6), 450–461.

Blacher, J., Cohen, S. R., & Azad, G. (2014). In the eye of the beholder: Reports of autism symptoms by Anglo and Latino mothers. *Research in Autism Spectrum Disorders, 8*(12), 1648–1656.

Blackwell, D. L., Martinez, M. E., Gentleman, J. F., Sanmartin, C., & Berthelot, J. M. (2009). Socioeconomic status and utilization of healthcare services in Canada and the United States: Findings from a binational healthcare survey. *Medical Care, 47*(11), 1136–1146.

Blair, I. V., Judd, C. M., & Fallman, J. L. (2004). The automaticity of race and Afrocentric facial features in social judgments. *Journal of Personality and Social Psychology, 87*, 763.

Boethel, M. (2003). *Diversity: School, family, and community connections. Annual synthesis 2003*. Austin, TX: National Center for Family and Community Schools, Southwest Educational Development Laboratory.

Borman, G. D., & Kimball, S. M. (2005). Teacher quality and educational equality: Do teachers with higher standards-based evaluation ratings close student achievement gaps? *The Elementary School Journal, 106*(1), 3–20.

Boss, R. D., Donohue, P. K., Larson, S. M., Arnold, R. M., & Roter, D. L. (2016). Family conferences in the neonatal intensive care unit: Observation of communication dynamics and contributions. *Pediatric Critical Care Medicine: A Journal of the Society of Critical Care Medicine and the World Federation of Pediatric Intensive and Critical Care Societies, 17*(3), 223.

Boulware, L., Cooper, L. A., Ratner, L. L., LaVeist, T., & Rowe, N. (2003). Race and trust in the health care system. *Public Health Reports, 118*, 358–365.

Boyd, B. A., & Correa, V. I. (2005). Developing a framework for reducing the cultural clash between African American parents and the special education system. *Multicultural Perspectives, 7*(2), 3–11.

Boyd, B. A., Odom, S. L., Humphreys, B. P., & Sam, A. M. (2010). Infants and toddlers with autism spectrum disorder: Early identification and early intervention. *Journal of Early Intervention, 32*(2), 75–98.

Burke, M. M., Goldman, S. E., Hart, M. S., & Hodapp, R. M. (2016). Evaluating the efficacy of a special education advocacy training program. *Journal of Policy and Practice in Intellectual Disabilities, 13*(4), 269–276.

Byington, T. A., & Whitby, P. J. S. (2011). Empowering families during the early intervention planning process. *Young Exceptional Children, 14*(4), 44–56.

Cai, X., Kaiser, A. P., & Hancock, T. B. (2004). Parent and teacher agreement on child behavior checklist items in a sample of preschoolers from low-income and predominantly African American families. *Journal of Clinical Child and Adolescent Psychology, 33*(2), 303–312.

Carr, T., & Lord, C. (2013). Longitudinal study of perceived negative impact in African American and Caucasian mothers of children with autism spectrum disorder. *Autism: the International Journal of Research and Practice, 17*(4), 405–417.

Cavaco, A., & Roter, D. (2010). Pharmaceutical consultations in community pharmacies: Utility of the roter interaction analysis system to study pharmacist–patient communication. *International Journal of Pharmacy Practice, 18*(3), 141–148.

Centers for Disease Control and Prevention. (2014). Prevalence of autism spectrum disorder among children aged 8 years — autism and developmental disabilities monitoring network, 11 sites, United States, 2010. *MMWR. Morbidity and Mortality Weekly Report, 63*(2), 1–22.

Childre, A., & Chambers, C. R. (2005). Family perceptions of student centered planning and IEP meetings. *Education and Training in Developmental Disabilities, 40*(3), 217–233.

Cooley, W. C., & Sagerman, P. J. (2011). Supporting the health care transition from adolescence to adulthood in the medical home. *Pediatrics, 128*(1), 182–200.

Cooper-Patrick, L., Gallo, J. J., Gonzales, J. J., Vu, H. T., Powe, N. R., Nelson, C., & Ford, D. E. (1999). Race, gender, and partnership in the patient-physician relationship. *Jama, 282*(6), 583–589.

Cooper, L. A., Roter, D., Bone, L., Larson, S. M., Miller, E. R., Barr, M., … Levine, D. M. (2009). A randomized controlled trial of interventions to enhance patient-physician partnership, patient adherence and high blood pressure control among ethnic minorities and poor persons. *Implementation Science, 4*, 1–16.

Cooper, L. A., Roter, D., Carson, K., Beach, M. C., Sabin, J., Greenwald, A., & Inui, T. S. (2012). The associations of clinicians' implicit attitudes about race with medical visit communication and patient ratings of interpersonal care. *American Journal of Public Health, 102*, 979–987.

Cooper, L. A., Roter, D. L., Carson, K. A., Bone, L. R., Larson, S. M., Miller, E. R., … Levine, D. M. (2011). A randomized trial to improve patient-centered care and hypertension control in underserved primary care patients. *Journal of General Internal Medicine, 26*(11), 1297–1304.

Cuccaro, M. L., Brinkley, J., Abramson, R. K., Hall, A., Wright, H. H., Hussman, J. P., … Pericak-Vance, M. A. (2007). Autism in African American families: Clinical-phenotypic findings. *American Journal of Medical Genetics B: Neuropsychiatric Genetics, 144B*(8), 1022–1026.

Darling-Hammond, L. (2004). Standards, accountability, and school reform. *Teachers College Record, 106*(6), 1047–1085. The Hammond 2004 is actually cited as Darling-Hammond 2004.

Dasgupta, N., & Greenwald, A. G. (2001). On the malleability of automatic attitudes: Combating automatic prejudice with images of admired and disliked individuals. *Journal of Personality and Social Psychology, 81*(5), 800.

Davis, J. E. (1983). *Professional and parent behavior at planning meetings related to a handicapped child's individualized educational plan.* Unpublished Manuscript.

Dhingra, S. S., Zack, M., Strine, T., Pearson, W. S., & Balluz, L. (2010). Determine prevalence and correlates of psychiatric treatment with Andersen's behavioral model of health services use. *Psychiatric Services, 61*(5), 524–528.

Dodge, K. A., Bai, Y., Ladd, H. F., & Muschkin, C. G. (2017). Impact of North Carolina's early childhood programs and policies on educational outcomes in elementary school. *Child Development, 88*(3), 996–1014. https://doi.org/10.1111/cdev.12645.

Dotterer, A. M., & Lowe, K. (2015). Perceived discrimination, parenting, and academic adjustment among racial/ethnic minority adolescents. *Journal of Applied Developmental Psychology, 41*, 71–77.

Dovidio, J. F., Kawakami, K., & Gaertner, S. L. (2002). Implicit and explicit prejudice and interracial interaction. *Journal of Personality and Social Psychology, 82*, 62.

Dunst, C. J., & Trivette, C. M. (1996). Empowerment, effective helpgiving practices and family- centered care. *Pediatric Nursing, 22*(4), 334–338.

Dunst, C. J., Trivette, C. M., & Hamby, D. W. (2007). Meta-analysis of family-centered helpgiving practices research. *Mental Retardation and Developmental Disabilities Research Reviews, 13*(4), 370–378.

Durkin, M. S., Maenner, M. J., Meaney, F. J., Levy, S. E., DiGuiseppi, C., Nicholas, J. S., & Schieve, L. A. (2010). Socioeconomic inequality in the prevalence of autism spectrum disorder: evidence from a US cross-sectional study. *PloS one, 5*(7), e11551.

Dworzynski, K., Ronald, A., Bolton, P., & Happé, F. (2012). How different are girls and boys above and below the diagnostic threshold for autism spectrum disorders? *Journal of the American Academy of Child and Adolescent Psychiatry, 51*(8), 788–797.

Entwisle, J. S., & Alexander, K. L. (1988). Factors affecting achievement test scores and marks of Black and White first graders. *The Elementary School Journal, 88*, 449–471.

Erevelles, N., & Minear, A. (2010). Unspeakable offenses: Untangling race and disability in discourses of intersectionality. *Journal of Literary & Cultural Disability Studies, 4*(2), 127–145.

Fountain, C., Winter, A. S., & Bearman, P. S. (2012). Six developmental trajectories characterize children with autism. *Pediatrics, peds-2011.*

Gartin, B. C., & Murdick, N. L. (2005). IDEA 2004: The IEP. *Remedial and Special Education, 26*(6), 327–331.

Gaskin, D. J., Zare, H., Haider, A. H., & LaVeist, T. A. (2016). The Quality of Surgical and Pneumonia Care in Minority-Serving and Racially Integrated Hospitals. *Health Services Research, 51*(3), 910–936.

Greenfield, D. B., Iruka, I. U., & Munis, P. (2004). Assessment of social competence in high-risk preschoolers: Evaluation of the adaptive social behavior inventory (ASBI) across home and school settings. *Journal of Psychoeducational Assessment, 22*(3), 220–232.

Greenwald, A. G., & Banaji, M. R. (1995). Implicit social cognition: Attitudes, self-esteem, and stereotypes. *Psychological Review, 102*(1), 4.

Greenwald, R., Hedges, L. V., & Laine, R. D. (1996). The effect of school resources on student achievement. *Review of educational research, 66*(3), 361–396.

Greenwald, A. G., McGhee, D. E., & Schwartz, J. L. (1998). Measuring individual differences in implicit cognition: The implicit association test. *Journal of Personality and Social Psychology, 74*(6), 1464.

Greenwood, C. R., Carta, J. J., Walker, D., Watson-Thompson, J., Gilkerson, J., Larson, A. L., & Schnitz, A. (2017). Conceptualizing a public health prevention intervention for bridging the 30 million word gap. *Clinical Child and Family Psychology Review, 20*(1), 3–24.

Gumperz, J. J., & Cook-Gumperz, J. (1981). *Ethnic differences in communicative style. Language in the USA.*

Hammond, W. P., Matthews, D., & Corbie-Smith, G. (2010). Psychosocial factors associated with routine health examination scheduling and receipt among African American men. *Journal of the National Medical Association, 102*(4), 276–289.

Harry, B., Allen, N., & McLaughlin, M. (1995). Communication versus compliance: African -American parents' involvement in special education. *Exceptional Children, 61*(4), 364–377.

Harry, B., & Anderson, M. G. (1994). The disproportionate placement of African American males in special education programs: A critique of the process. *The Journal of Negro Education, 63*(4), 602–619.

Haveman, R., & Wolfe, B. (1995). The determinants of children's attainments: A review of methods and findings. *Journal of Economic Literature, 33*(4), 1829–1878.

Hill, N. E., Castellino, D. R., Lansford, J. E., Nowlin, P., Dodge, K. A., Bates, J. E., & Pettit, G. S. (2004). Parent academic involvement as related to school behavior, achievement, and aspirations: Demographic variations across adolescence. *Child Development, 75*(5), 1491–1509.

Hughes, J. N., Gleason, K. A., & Zhang, D. (2005). Relationship influences on teachers' perceptions of academic competence in academically at-risk minority and majority first grade students. *Journal of School Psychology, 43*(4), 303–320.

Hughes, J., & Oi-man, K. (2007). Influence of student-teacher and parent-teacher relationships on lower achieving readers' engagement and achievement in the primary grades. *Journal of Educational Psychology, 99*, 39–51.
Individuals with Disabilities Education Improvement Act of 2004, P.L. 108-446, 20 U.S.C. $ 1400 et seq.
Insaf, T. Z., Jurkowski, J. M., & Alomar, L. (2010). Sociocultural factors influencing delay in seeking routine healthcare among Latinas. A community-based participatory research study. *Ethnicity & Disease, 20*(2), 148–154.
Iruka, I. U., Dotterer, A. M., & Pungello, E. P. (2014). Ethnic variations of pathways linking socioeconomic status, parenting, and preacademic skills in a nationally representative sample. *Early Education & Development, 25*(7), 973–994. https://doi.org/10.1080/10409289.2014.892806.
Iruka, I. U., LaForett, D. R., & Odom, E. C. (2012). Examining the validity of the family investment and stress models and relationship to children's school readiness across five cultural groups. *Journal of Family Psychology, 26*(3), 359–370. https://doi.org/10.1037/a0028290.
Iruka, I. U., Winn, D.-M. C., Kingsley, S. J., & Orthodoxou, Y. J. (2011). Links between parent -teacher relationships and kindergartners' social skills: Do ethnicity and family income matter? *The Elementary School Journal, 111*(3), 387–408.
Irvin, D. W., McBee, M., Boyd, B. A., Hume, K., & Odom, S. L. (2012). Child and family factors associated with the use of services for preschoolers with autism spectrum disorder. *Research in Autism Spectrum Disorders, 6*(1), 565–572.
Jeffries, M., & Grogan, S. (2012). 'Oh, I'm just, you know, a little bit weak because I'm going to the doctor's': Young men's talk of self-referral to primary healthcare services. *Psychology and Health, 27*(8), 898–915.
Jiang, Y., Granja, M. R., & Koball, H. (2017). Basic Facts about Low-Income Children: Children under 6 Years, 2015. Fact Sheet. *National Center for Children in Poverty.*
Jo Landmark, L., Zhang, D. D., & Montoya, L. (2007). Culturally diverse parents' experiences in their children's transition: Knowledge and involvement. *Career Development for Exceptional Individuals, 30*(2), 68–79.
Johnson, R. L., Roter, D., Powe, N. R., & Cooper, L. A. (2004). Patient race/ethnicity and quality of patient-physician communication during medical visits. *American Journal of Public Health, 94*, 2084–2090.
Kaplan, S. H., Greenfield, S., & Ware, J. E., Jr. (1989). Assessing the effects of physician-patient interactions on the outcomes of chronic disease. *Medical Care*, S110–S127.
Kilbourne, A. M., Switzer, G., Hyman, K., Crowley-Matoka, M., & Fine, M. (2006). Advancing health disparities research within the health care system: A conceptual framework. *American Journal of Public Health, 96*, 2113–2121.
Kochhar-Bryant, C. A., & Izzo, M. V. (2006). Access to post-high school services: Transition assessment and the summary of performance. *Career Development for Exceptional Individuals, 29*(2), 70–89.
Kogan, M. D., Blumberg, S. J., Schieve, L. A., Boyle, C. A., Perrin, J. M., Ghandour, R. M., … van Dyck, P. C. (2009). Prevalence of parent-reported diagnosis of autism spectrum disorder among children in the US, 2007. *Pediatrics, 124*(5), 1395–1403.
Kuppens, T., & Spears, R. (2014). You don't have to be well-educated to be an aversive racist, but it helps. *Social Science Research, 45*, 211–223.
La Vonne, I. N., McCray, A. D., Webb-Johnson, G., & Bridgest, S. T. (2003). The effects of African American movement styles on teachers' perceptions and reactions. *The Journal of Special Education, 37*(1), 49–57.

Lamb-Parker, F., Piotrkowski, C. S., Baker, A. J. L., Kessler-Sklar, S., Clark, B., & Peay, L. (2001). Understanding barriers to parent involvement in Head start: A research -community partnership. *Early Childhood Research Quarterly, 16*(1), 35–51.
Lee, B. K., & McGrath, J. J. (2015). Advancing parental age and autism: Multifactorial pathways. *Trends in Molecular Medicine, 21*(2), 118–125.
Little, P., Everitt, H., Williamson, I., Warner, G., Moore, M., Gould, C., ... Payne, S. (2001). Observational study of effect of patient centredness and positive approach on outcomes of general practice consultations. *Bmj: British Medical Journal, 323*(7318), 908–911.
Liptak, G. S., Benzoni, L. B., Mruzek, D. W., Nolan, K. W., Thingvoll, M. A., Wade, C. M., & Fryer, G. E. (2008). Disparities in diagnosis and access to health services for children with autism: data from the National Survey of Children's Health. *Journal of Developmental & Behavioral Pediatrics, 29*(3), 152–160.
Lynch, E. C., & Beare, P. L. (1990). The quality of IEP objectives and their relevance to instruction for students with mental retardation and behavioral disorders. *Remedial and Special Education, 11*(2), 48–55.
Magaña, S., Parish, S. L., Rose, R. A., Timberlake, M., & Swaine, J. G. (2012). Racial and ethnic disparities in quality of health care among children with autism and other developmental disabilities. *Intellectual and developmental disabilities, 50*(4), 287–299.
Mandell, D. S., Listerud, J., Levy, S. E., & Pinto-Martin, J. A. (2002). Race differences in the age at diagnosis among Medicaid-eligible children with autism. *Journal of the American Academy of Child & Adolescent Psychiatry, 41*(12), 1447–1453.
Mandell, D. S., & Novak, M. (2005). The role of culture in families' treatment decisions for children with autism spectrum disorder. *Mental Retardation and Developmental Disabilities Research Reviews, 11*, 110–115.
Mandell, D. S., Wiggins, L. D., Carpenter, L. A., Daniels, J., DiGuiseppi, C., Durkin, M. S., ... Kirby, R. S. (2009). Racial/ethnic disparities in the identification of children with autism spectrum disorders. *American Journal of Public Health, 99*(3), 493–498.
Manning, M. M., Wainwright, L., & Bennett, J. (2011). The double ABCX model of adaptation in racially diverse families with a school-age child with autism. *Journal of Autism and Developmental Disorders, 41*(3), 320–331.
Mehta, N. K., Lee, H., & Ylitalo, K. R. (2013). Child health in the United States: Recent trends in racial/ethnic disparities. *Social Science & Medicine, 95*, 6–15.
Meyers, M. K., & Jordan, L. P. (2006). Choice and accommodation in parental child care decisions. *Community Development, 37*(2), 53–70.
Mistry, R. S., Biesanz, J. C., Chien, N., Howes, C., & Benner, A. D. (2008). Socioeconomic status, parental investments, and the cognitive and behavioral outcomes of low-income children from immigrant and native households. *Early Childhood Research Quarterly, 23*(2), 193–212.
New York Appleseed, n.d. *New York city elementary schools: A tale of two cities*. New York, NY: Author.
Nosek, B. A., Banaji, M., & Greenwald, A. G. (2002). Harvesting implicit group attitudes and beliefs from a demonstration web site. *Group Dynamics: Theory, Research, and Practice, 6*(1), 101.
Okonofua, J. A., & Eberhardt, J. L. (2015). Two strikes race and the disciplining of young students. *Psychological Science, 26*(5), 617–624.
O'Connor, C., & Fernandez, S. D. (2006). Race, class, and disproportionality: Reevaluating the relationship between poverty and special education placement. *Educational Researcher, 35*(6), 6–11.

Penner, L. A., Dovidio, J. F., West, T. V., Gaertner, S. L., Albrecht, T. L., Dailey, R. K., & Markova, T. (2010). Aversive racism and medical interactions with Black patients: A field study. *Journal of Experimental Social Psychology, 46*, 436–440.

Phillips, K. A., Morrison, K. R., Andersen, R., & Aday, L. A. (1998). Understanding the context of healthcare utilization: Assessing environmental and provider-related variables in the behavioral model of utilization. *Health Services Research, 33*(3), 571–596.

Rachlinski, J. J., Johnson, S. L., Wistrich, A. J., & Guthrie, C. (2009). Does unconscious racial bias affect trial judges? *The Notre Dame Law Review, 84*, 09–11.

Rai, D., Lewis, G., Lundberg, M., Araya, R., Svensson, A., Dalman, C., & Magnusson, C. (2012). Parental socioeconomic status and risk of offspring autism spectrum disorders in a Swedish population-based study. *Journal of the American Academy of Child & Adolescent Psychiatry, 51*(5), 467–476.

Raver, C. C., Gershoff, E. T., & Aber, J. L. (2007). Testing equivalence of mediating models of income, parenting, and school readiness for White, Black, and Hispanic children in a national sample. *Child Development, 78*(1), 96–115.

Reardon, S. F. (2016). School segregation and racial achievement gaps. *Russell Sage Foundation Journal of the Social Sciences, 2*(5), 34–57.

Reardon, S. F., & Fahle, E. M. (2017). Education. In *State of the Union: The poverty and inequality report* (pp. 20–23). Stanford, CA: Stanford Center on Poverty and Inequality.

Roter, D. L., & Hall, J. A. (1992). *Doctors talking with patients/patients talking with doctors: Improving communication in medical visits*. Westport, CT: Auburn House.

Roter, D. L., & Larson, S. (2001). The relationship between residents' and attending physicians' communication during primary care visits: An illustrative use of the Roter Interaction Analysis System. *Journal of Health Communication, 13*(1), 33–48.

Ruble, L., McGrew, J., Dalrymple, N., & Jung, L. (2010). Examining the quality of IEPs for young children with autism. *Journal of Autism and Developmental Disorders, 40*(12), 1459–1470.

Rumberger, R. W., & Palardy, G. J. (2005). Does segregation still matter? The impact of student composition on academic achievement in high school. *Teachers college record, 107*(9), 1999.

Ruppar, A. L., & Gaffney, J. S. (2011). Individualized education program team decisions: A preliminary study of conversations, negotiations, and power. *Research and Practice for Persons with Severe Disabilities, 36*(1/2), 11–22.

Shattuck, P. T., Wagner, M., Narendorf, S., Sterzing, P., & Hensley, M. (2011). Post–high school service use among young adults with an autism spectrum disorder. *Archives of pediatrics & adolescent medicine, 165*(2), 141–146.

Staats, C., & Patton, C. (2013). State of the science: Implicit bias review 2013. *Kirwan Institute for the Study of Race and Ethnicity, 14*, 129–142.

Stewart, M. A. (1995). Effective physician-patient communication and health outcomes: A review. *Journal of the Canadian Medical Association, 152*(9), 1423–1433.

Tek, S., & Landa, R. J. (2012). Differences in autism symptoms between minority and non-minority toddlers. *Journal of autism and developmental disorders, 42*(9), 1967–1973.

Thomas, K. C., Ellis, A. R., McLaurin, C., Daniels, J., & Morrissey, J. P. (2007). Access to care for autism-related services. *Journal of autism and developmental disorders, 37*(10), 1902–1912.

Thornton, R. L. J., Powe, N. R., Roter, D., & Cooper, L. A. (2011). Patient–physician social concordance, medical visit communication and patients' perceptions of health care quality. *Patient Education and Counseling, 85*(3), e201–e208.

Van den Bergh, L., Denessen, E., Hornstra, L., Voeten, M., & Holland, R. W. (2010). The implicit prejudiced attitudes of teachers relations to teacher expectations and the ethnic achievement gap. *American Educational Research Journal, 47*(2), 497–527.

Viele, M. K., & Weiskopf, R. B. (1994). What can we learn about the need for transfusion from patients who refuse blood? The experience with Jehovah's Witnesses. *Transfusion, 34*(5), 396–401.
Williams, D. R., & Jackson, P. B. (2005). Social sources of racial disparities in health. *Health affairs, 24*(2), 325–334.
Wong, S. W., & Hughes, J. N. (2006). Ethnicity and language contributions to dimensions of parent involvement. *School Psychology Review, 35*(4), 645–662.
Ziegert, J. C., & Hanges, P. J. (2005). Employment discrimination: The role of implicit attitudes, motivation, and a climate for racial bias. *Journal of Applied Psychology, 90*, 553.

CHAPTER TWO

Family-Professional Partnerships With Refugee Families of Children With Disabilities

Shana J. Haines*[,1], Grace L. Francis[§], Kathleen B. Kyzar[¶], Heather M. Aldersey[||] and Nicole B. Adams[#]
*University of Vermont, Burlington, VT, United States
[§]George Mason University, Fairfax, VA, United States
[¶]Texas Christian University, Fort Worth, TX, United States
[||]Queen's University, Kingston, ON, Canada
[#]University of Illinois, Urbana-Champaign, IL, United States
[1]Corresponding Author: E-mail: Shana.haines@uvm.edu

Contents

Abstract

Research demonstrates the positive impact of family-professional partnerships on student and family outcomes. Despite the importance of family-professional partnerships, however, research on such partnerships with refugee families of children with disabilities has been largely absent from the research literature. The aim of this article is to review existing research regarding building and maintaining partnerships between refugee families and school professionals for refugees who have been resettled to host countries, or countries that grant refugees legal status as permanent residents. We discuss implications for U.S. educational systems and offer recommendations for future research.

International Review of Research in Developmental Disabilities, Volume 54
ISSN 2211-6095
https://doi.org/10.1016/bs.irrdd.2018.07.002

Successful schools ensure that all students and their families are valued members of the school community (Francis, Blue-Banning, Haines, Turnbull, & Gross, 2016) and provide environments where all students, families, and teachers feel that they belong (Foley et al., 2012). Strong family-professional partnerships are imperative to these successful schools (Francis et al., 2016). Family-professional partnerships occur when families and education professionals regard each other as reliable allies, and education professionals provide families with multiple opportunities for meaningful participation in their children's education (Haines, McCart, & Turnbull, 2013). Research demonstrates the positive impact of family-professional partnerships on student and family outcomes and documents numerous strategies for their implementation (Bryan & Henry, 2012; Henderson & Mapp, 2002; Tschannen-Moran, 2014). Such strategies include forming positive and trusting relationships, outlining clear roles and responsibilities, engaging in ongoing communication, identifying shared resources, acknowledging mutual goals, demonstrating professional competency, and building family leadership (Francis et al., 2016; Tonelson & Waters, 1993). It is imperative that all students and their families, including diverse and historically marginalized populations, are considered valued members of the school community.

Despite the importance of family-professional partnerships for positive school and stakeholder outcomes, historically marginalized families of children with disabilities, including immigrant and refugee families, face many systemic barriers related to developing partnerships with educators. Such barriers include school professionals carrying out microaggressions against students/families and holding stereotypical or discriminatory views (Cooper, Riehl, & Hasan, 2010; Dávila, 2015; Francis, Gross, Lavin, Casarez, & Sheets, 2018; Harry, 2008). Families from historically marginalized populations often lack access to interpreters and translated documents (Francis et al., 2018; Pang, 2011) and infrequently receive resources and services that are appropriate for meeting their needs (Gothberg, Greene, & Kohler, 2018). Finally, both families and educators from these groups report that they are unprepared to effectively collaborate (Landmark, Roberts, & Zhang, 2013). It is not surprising that these barriers exist given the dearth of research on partnership practices specific to refugee families of children with disabilities, and strengthening family-professional partnerships with this population is of utmost importance due to their unfamiliarity with the American special education system and knowledge of family rights and responsibilities (Francis, Haines, & Nagro, 2017; Haines & Francis, 2016).

The purpose of this article is to review existing research regarding building and maintaining partnerships between refugee families of children with disabilities and school professionals, with the aim of drawing implications from this review to enhance partnerships in U.S. schools and to define a research agenda to strengthen the field in this topic. To our knowledge, this review represents the first attempt at systematically locating and synthesizing research related to family-professional partnerships within special education that is specific to refugee populations. We focus on research involving refugee populations who are in host countries of resettlement, or countries that grant refugees legal status as permanent residents such as the U.S., Canada, New Zealand, and Australia, in order to determine its application to practice in the U.S.

This article weaves together five major topics. We first define the term "refugee" and provide background on refugee populations living in the U.S. Second, we discuss why the topic of family-professional partnerships is important, especially for refugee populations. Third, we outline the Sunshine Model (Haines et al., 2017), a framework for conceptualizing family-professional partnerships. Fourth, we discuss the existing research on family-professional partnerships with refugee families of children with disabilities in host countries of resettlement. Finally, we discuss implications for future research and practice in U.S. schools.

1. REFUGEES IN THE U.S.

At the end of 2016, violence and persecution had forced 65.5 million people from their homes (UNHCR, 2017), including 10.3 million people newly displaced during that year alone. Of these, 40.3 million were internally-displaced people (i.e., people who left their homes to flee conflict but have not crossed a border into another country); 17.2 million were asylum-seekers (i.e., people who requested sanctuary but are still waiting to receive it); and 22.5 million people were refugees, the highest number on record. The 1951 Convention Relating to the Status of Refugees defined a refugee as:

> *[A person who,] owing to wellfounded fear of being persecuted for reasons of race, religion, nationality, membership of a particular social group or political opinion, is outside the country of his [sic] nationality and is unable or, owing to such fear, is unwilling to avail himself [sic] of the protection of that country; or who, not having a nationality and being outside the country of his [sic] former habitual residence as a result of such events, is unable or, owing to such fear, is unwilling to return to it.*
>
> ***UNHCR (2010)***

Of the 22.5 million refugees recorded in 2016, 552,200 have returned home, 189,300 were resettled in a host country, and the remainder are living in countries of asylum (UNHCR, 2017). The U.S. resettled the highest number of refugees in 2016, at 96,900, followed by Canada (46,700), and Australia (27,600; UNHCR, 2017). Refugees were resettled from Syria (63,000), Democratic Republic of the Congo (22,100), Iraq (14,700), Somalia (12,200), and in smaller numbers from other countries (e.g., Burma, Ukraine, Bhutan, Iran, Eritrea; UNHCR, 2017). The recent war in Syria, currently in its seventh year, has resulted in millions of people living in fear and lacking access to education, food, and healthcare (UNHCR, 2018a). In Congo, the eastern regions continue to be devastated by decades of unrest following a brutal civil war in the 1990s. Many people have returned home to find their communities and schools in ruins; mutilation, sexual violence, and murder continue in this region (UNHCR, 2018b).

1.1 Refugee Resettlement

The process of refugee resettlement to the U.S., from filing the initial paperwork for resettlement to landing in their new country, can be long and arduous, averaging 18–24 months (U.S. Bureau of Population, Refugees, and Migration, 2018). This process involves intense scrutiny to ensure that an individual seeking refugee status qualifies as a refugee by having a well-founded fear of persecution based on religion, political opinion, race, nationality, or membership in a particular social group. Once the threat of persecution is established and it is determined that the refugee cannot return home or settle in the country of asylum, the United Nations High Commissioner for Refugees (UNHCR) refers them for resettlement. Only about 1% of refugees are resettled in a host country. Family ties, language ability, and professional skills help determine in which country an individual will be resettled (U.S. Committee for Refugees and Immigrants, n.d.). UNHCR then refers refugees to host countries (keeping families together to the greatest extent possible). In the case of the U.S., the U.S. Refugee Resettlement Program oversees the process by which refugees undergo intense security screening. Once approved for resettlement in the U.S., refugees are matched with one of 11 designated non-governmental agencies, such as the U.S. Committee for Refugees and Immigrants or World Relief, that aid them in resettlement. Prior to the refugees' arrival in the U.S., the agencies receive federal funding to aid refugees in resettlement in their host country. While still in the country of asylum, agency employees assist refugees to complete paperwork, provide assessments leading to requisite medical clearances, and provide a cultural orientation aimed at teaching basic information about the resettlement process in the U.S., including expectations for self-sufficiency. Refugees sign promissory notes agreeing to repay the U.S. government for all travel costs ensued by their journey to their new country (U.S. Committee for Refugees and Immigrants, n.d.).

When resettled refugees arrive in the U.S. as permanent residents, the resettlement agency to which they have been assigned helps them settle in and acclimate to their new communities (U.S. Department of State, n.d.). Agency staff meet refugees at the airport, provide a safe and affordable place for them to stay, and help take care of their needs for at least 90 days after arrival (U.S. Committee for Refugees and Immigrants, n.d.). Typical supports include helping them apply for a Social Security number, registering children for school, arranging medical evaluations, enrolling adults in English language training, and helping adults find employment (U.S. Committee for Refugees and Immigrants, n.d.).

Encountering education systems. Enrolling students in school is of utmost importance to many refugee families (Atwell, Gifford, & McDonald-Wilmsen, 2009; Schiller, Boggis, Messenger, & Douglas, 2009). In fact, one of the most important reasons for resettling to a host country is a quality education as many refugee families were not able to consistently access this for their children before resettlement (McBrien, 2011). The U.S. education systems contrasts greatly with education systems of countries of origin (Atwell et al., 2009; Hwa-Froelich & Westby, 2003; Tadesse, Hoot, & Watson-Thompson, 2009), and sometimes specific populations, like the Somali Bantu, had no access to education before resettlement (Birman & Tran, 2015). Three of the most salient educational differences between host countries and countries of origin are (a) the role and responsibility of families in working with teachers to educate students (i.e., different expectations of family-professional partnerships; Haines, Summers, Turnbull, & Turnbull, 2015a; He, Bettez, & Levin, 2017; Isik-Ercan, 2012; McBrien, 2011; Miller-Gairy & Mofya, 2015; Tadesse, 2014), (b) pedagogy and behavior management techniques (Birman & Tran, 2015; Haines et al., 2015a,b; Tadesse, Hoot, & Watson-Thomas, 2009), and (c) the meaning of disability and how it affects a student's educability (Kalyanpur & Harry, 2012).

Families' perceptions of their roles and the roles of teachers in educating children may differ from the teachers' perceptions of these roles (He et al., 2017). Many refugee families draw a line between school and home, perceiving teachers' roles and responsibilities as ensuring children learn academics, and the family and community responsibilities as ensuring children's moral and cultural upbringing (Isik-Ercan, 2012). Furthermore, some refugee families prefer entrusting teachers to educate their children; they do not want to meddle with their child's education, as it is a process about which they feel they know little (Haines et al., 2015a; Isik-Ercan, 2012). This belief, in general, is undergirded by the fact that some refugee families have low levels of education and do not believe that they could help educate their children. These families might also have very low expectations for family-professional partnerships because they have never experienced them (Haines, Summers, Turnbull, Palmer, & Turnbull, 2015b).

In turn, these role perceptions may be compounded by families' unfamiliarity with the pedagogy and systems found in American schools (Birman, Trickett, & Bacchus, 2001; Dachyshyn & Kirova, 2008; Tadesse et al., 2009; Walker-Dalhouse & Dalhouse, 2009), such as constructivist or experiential teaching, proficiency-based learning, special education, and related arts. Refugee families may have different expectations for their children's behavior than teachers, which can cause confusion and potentially result in families distancing themselves from school even more (Haines et al., 2015a; Hurley, Medici, Stewart, & Cohen, 2011; Tadesse et al., 2009; Walker-Dalhouse & Dalhouse, 2009). Furthermore, disability in many cultures is perceived as rendering a child uneducable (Aldersey & Haines, 2017), and many families do not consider sending their children with disabilities to school or have high expectations for them (Kalyanpur & Harry, 2012). In this article, we primarily focus on the intersection of these areas of contrast: family-professional partnerships for refugee families of children with disabilities.

2. FAMILY-PROFESSIONAL PARTNERSHIPS

Strong family-professional partnerships contribute to student success and, ultimately, to an equitable and democratic community (Skrtic, Sailor, & Gee, 1996), especially in schools with diverse populations (Leonard, 2011). Family-professional partnerships can also benefit all members of a school community—educators, families, and students (Henderson & Mapp, 2002). For students, family-professional partnerships have been linked with improvements in their behavior and increased attendance (Bryan & Henry, 2012; Ferguson, 2008; Giovacco-Johnson, 2009; Goddard, Tschannen-Moran, & Hoy, 2001; Lawson, 2003). Partnerships can also ensure that educational programming is culturally relevant (Kalyanpur & Harry, 2012). In addition, family-professional partnerships contribute to reduced levels of parental stress (Burke & Hodapp, 2014) by boosting family satisfaction, understanding, social connections, development, and parenting skills (Blue-Banning, Summers, Frankland, Nelson, & Beegle, 2004; Hill & Taylor, 2004). Stronger family-professional partnerships are also correlated with increased family quality of life (Eskow, Summers, Cahsson, & Mitchell, 2018; Kyzar, Brady, Summers, Haines, & Turnbull, 2016). Further, family-professional partnerships are linked with increased educator skill and effectiveness and stronger relationships among community members (Hill & Taylor, 2004; Lawson, 2003). Moreover, family-professional partnerships are related to trust among the greater school community, an outcome that leads to increased collective efficacy, academic optimism, and student achievement (Hoy, 2012).

Both general and special education policies in the U.S. underscore the need for relationships with families. U.S. special education, authorized by the Individuals with Disabilities Education Act (IDEA, 2004), is built on the premise that partnerships between parents and educators result in more effective educational programming leading to the four outcomes of disability policy: equal opportunity, economic self-sufficiency, full participation, and independent living (IDEA, 2004). IDEA grants parents the right to collaborate in making educational decisions, but this right comes with the expectation that families will partner with educational professionals to determine their children's educational needs and programs (Turnbull, Stowe, & Huerta, 2007). This policy assumes that parents understand and practice their legal rights and have the skills to be active advocates for their children with disabilities (Phillips, 2008).

The Every Student Succeeds Act (ESSA, 2015) also includes provisions related to family-professional partnerships that relate to all students, including those who do and do not qualify for special education services under IDEA. ESSA calls for "meaningful involvement" [Sec.1116(a)(2)(D)] for families who are "economically disadvantaged, are disabled, have limited English proficiency, have limited literacy, or of any racial or ethnic minority background" [Sec.1116(a)(2)(D)(i)] through implementing effective family outreach efforts, distributing written parent and family engagement policies, supporting educators to engage with families through knowledge sharing, and conducting annual assessments of school engagement efforts. ESSA also requires "ensuring regular two-way, meaningful communication between family members and school staff, and, to the extent practicable, in a language that family members can understand" [Sec.1116(d)(2)(D)]. IDEA and ESSA demonstrate that the U.S. government is seeking to build educational systems characterized by effective family-professional partnerships (Francis et al., 2018).

Despite policies and research clearly underscoring the importance of family-professional partnerships, research suggests that the realities of partnerships in the U.S. generally fall short (Blackwell & Rossetti, 2014; Haines et al., 2015a; LaRocque, Kleiman, & Darling, 2011; Mandic, Rudd, Hehir, & Acevedo-Garcia, 2012). The shortcoming in practice is due largely to differing conceptualizations of family-professional partnerships (Lawson, 2003), a lack of trust between families and professionals (LaRocque et al., 2011; Mapp & Hong, 2010), negative assumptions about the other party involved in partnerships (Haines & Reyes, 2018; Kalyanpur & Harry, 2012; Lea, 2006), and competing demands on educator time (Haines et al., 2015a,b). Additionally, families' beliefs about their roles in their children's education can greatly affect their partnerships with their children's teachers (Whitaker & Hoover-Dempsey, 2013). Whitaker and Hoover-Dempsey (2013) conducted a survey study aimed at examining links between parents' role beliefs for family-professional partnerships and variables contributing to its development. In the survey, 249 parents from two middle schools serving low-income students assessed their perceptions of student and teacher invitations to involvement, school expectations of involvement, school climate, their own childhood schooling experiences, and their role beliefs. Findings indicated that parents' perceptions of their child's interest in their involvement in school, school expectations of involvement, and school climate had the largest effects on parents' role beliefs.

These findings have strong implications for schools that serve resettled refugee populations. In such communities, families are learning about the school systems of their new countries and have usually experienced different expectations of relationships with teachers as well as notions of disability and educability in their regions of origin (Kalyanpur & Harry, 2012; Minhas, 2014; Yohani, 2013). Unfortunately, there is a notable paucity of research about family-professional partnerships between refugee families and professionals at their children's schools (Haines & Francis, 2016). The limited research that exists largely focuses on difficulties impeding the formation of family-professional partnerships for refugee families whose children attend school in the U.S.

2.1 Barriers to Partnerships Between Refugee Families and School Professionals

Numerous barriers to partnerships between refugee families and their children's teachers exist. First, professionals are often not knowledgeable about implementing research-based partnership strategies or identify partnering with families as a challenge (Epstein & Sanders, 2006; Markow, Macia, & Lee, 2013). These educators are even less prepared to partner with refugee families (Hurley, Saini, Warren, & Carberry, 2013; Hurley, Clark, Fonseca-Foster, Pyne, & Warren, 2017). Results of a recent national survey of 113 faculty members instructing in U.S. university-based special education programs revealed that only one-third of the participants included content specific to immigrant and/or refugee families in their non-partnership-specific courses (e.g., assessment course, instructional methods course; Kyzar, Mueller, Francis, & Haines, 2018). Because the data Kyzar et al. (2018) reported combined immigrant and refugee families, the proportion of the faculty participants who covered refugee populations specifically is, presumably, markedly lower.

Multiple other barriers to creating partnerships between refugee families of children with disabilities and their children's teachers are possible. Communication is key to creating partnerships, and language differences and varying literacy levels cause families and professionals to rely on interpreters or liaisons to interact with teachers (Atwell et al., 2009; Hurley et al., 2017; McBrien, 2005, 2011; Perry, 2009; Yohani, 2013). It can be difficult for families and teachers to access trained interpreters in a timely manner (Hurley et al., 2011). In addition, procedural safeguards are typically written at a 16th grade level in English (Mandic, Rudd, Hedir, & Acevedo-Garcia, 2012), and they are often not available in the languages refugees speak and read (e.g., Arabic, Maay—Maay, Somali, Swahili, Karen, Nepali). Other systemic issues, such as a lack of transportation and childcare as well as inflexible work hours for refugee families, can make forming partnerships difficult (Isik-Ercan, 2012).

Moreover, as discussed previously, refugee families may not have the desire to form such partnerships with teachers. Some may have a deference to professionals that hinders the formation of equal and reciprocal partnerships because such an attitude is inherent to hierarchical educational systems in their countries of origin (Jegatheesan, 2009; Lo, 2012; Whitaker & Hoover-Dempsey, 2013). Refugee families may view their role in educating their children differently from that expected by teachers

(Haines et al., 2015b; Isik-Ercan, 2012) due to their experiences, beliefs, and/or lack of confidence (Birman et al., 2001; Dachyshyn & Kirova, 2008; Tadesse et al., 2009; Walker-Dalhouse & Dalhouse, 2009). Misunderstanding or disagreement related to behavior expectations and management techniques may also affect family-professional partnerships (Hurley et al., 2011; Tadesse et al., 2009; Walker-Dalhouse & Dalhouse, 2009). In addition, a desire to keep private family information that could be stigmatizing or cause difficulty for the family may also affect refugee families' desire to partner with professionals (Jegatheesan, 2009; Tryer & Fazel, 2014; Walick & Sullivan, 2015). While many of the aforementioned challenges may be experienced by other cultural groups, refugee families experience more of a disadvantage due to the compounded nature of their beliefs and cultural experiences paired with personal histories of trauma, health concerns, and instability.

Clearly, there is a strong need to create family-professional partnerships for refugee families as well as many potential barriers to the creation of these relationships. A comprehensive model of family-professional partnerships can guide the examination of practice and research. Therefore, before examining the research that exists on this topic, we turn to such a model.

2.2 The Sunshine Model

A necessary step in narrowing the gap between the vision of family-professional partnerships articulated in policy and the reality of the field is to use a framework to guide research, policy, and practice. Haines et al. (2017) created the Sunshine Model for this purpose (see Fig. 1).

Forming trusting family-professional partnerships that enhance child, family, teacher, and system outcomes is the goal of the Sunshine Model, which is why it is in the center of the sun. The sun in the middle of the figure represents the power families and professionals have when they work together in all settings. This "solar power" (Turnbull & Turnbull, 2017) enables growth, warmth, and sustainability for all involved, helping foster the growth of the focal people as well as those who support them. The Sunshine Model aims to strengthen family-professional partnerships to foster collective power, trust, and reciprocity between families and professionals.

This model is based on principles of partnership, or the "how" of family-professional partnerships, and proactively establishes the activities typically conducted within the context of these relationships, or the "what" of family-professional partnerships. The principles of partnership include

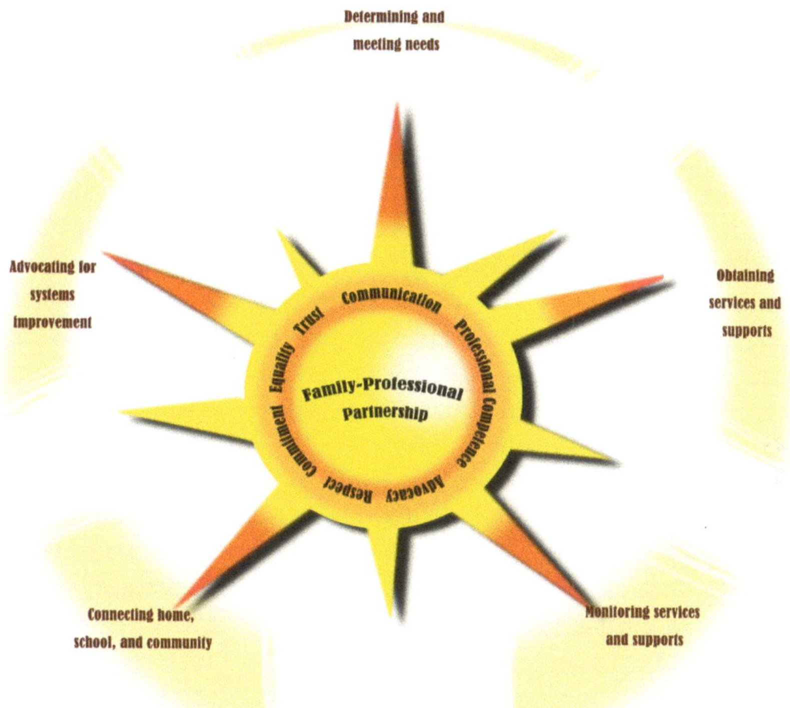

Figure 1 The Sunshine Model of family-professional partnerships (Haines et al., 2017). The Sunshine Model strengthens family-professional partnerships by elucidating the main principles of strong partnerships and the activities done through partnerships that foster collective power, trust, and reciprocity between families and professionals.

communication, respect, professional competence, commitment, equality, advocacy, and trust (Turnbull, Turnbull, Erwin, Soodak, & Shogren, 2015). Turnbull et al. (2015) liken these seven principles to a mobile, stating that "Without one of them, the others would not 'hang together' as well as they do" (p. 163). These principles result in forming trusting relationships through which to collaborate towards the five main activity types of family-professional partnerships.

The "partnership activities" are located towards the tips of the sun's rays. These activity types include (a) determining and meeting needs; (b) obtaining services and supports; (c) monitoring services and supports; (d) connecting home, school, and community; and (e) advocating for systems improvement. These activity types are specific enough to enable proactive discussion, planning, and conceptualizing, yet they are intentionally broad enough to be responsive to the fluid needs of individual families within the unique context of their schools and communities. Considering these partnership activities can be instructive in addressing the barriers to partnership discussed above.

The Sunshine Model is conceptualized to flexibly respond to all families and students based on open and reciprocal communication between educators and families to determine needs and strategies. Tiers or intensity of support for family-professional partnerships appear in the Sunshine Model within the rays of sunshine representing the types of activities done in partnership (Haines et al., 2017). The Sunshine Model's broadness enables it to be operationalized in ways that are responsive to the fluid needs of specific families, schools, and communities. In focusing comprehensively on both the "how" and the "what" of family-professional partnerships, the Sunshine Model is helpful for deeply examining many aspects of practice and research involving historically marginalized or disenfranchised families, such as refugee families. In the following section, we use the Sunshine Model as an organizational structure through which to review research pertaining to family-professional partnerships specific to refugee families of children with disabilities.

3. SHINING A LIGHT ON THE RESEARCH LANDSCAPE

This review is the first article that synthesizes research related to family-professional partnerships with refugee families whose children have disabilities. It is focused specifically on research within refugee populations because this heterogeneous population is bound by their requisite experience of being uprooted, fleeing persecution, and having little if any input into their location of resettlement. Most refugees come to the U.S. seeking a more stable life for themselves and their children—one that is safe and free from oppression. Many refugees find themselves resettled to mid-sized cities throughout the U.S. that do not have sizeable immigrant populations other than refugees (Bernstein & Dubois, 2018). Schools in such communities may not be equipped to work with refugees, especially when the countries of origin and language of the refugee populations change frequently (Hurley et al., 2011). Educators in such communities often do not have extensive experience working with families from such diverse backgrounds. Systems that are not established to proactively partner with refugee families coupled with educators who do not have the knowledge and skills to partner with these families impede refugee families' abilities to help their children succeed in school. Further, the expectation of family-professional partnerships inherent in U.S. educational systems, especially when the children have disabilities or struggle with school, must be modeled and explained in order for refugee families to fully understand the potential shift to the roles and responsibilities inherent in U.S. schools. These factors warrant the study of refugee populations in general and those whose children have disabilities in particular. Gathering a comprehensive portrayal of research pertaining to family-professional partnerships for refugee families of children with disabilities and who are resettled in host countries is complicated, however.

A barrier to gaining a comprehensive understanding of the research on family-professional partnership with refugee families of children with disabilities is the term *refugee*. A refugee is a specific type of immigrant, and, for various reasons, this term is not often used as a keyword, in the title, or in the abstract of articles. One reason for this is because, in accordance with IDEA regulations and Plyler v. Doe (1982) determinations, public sector professionals (e.g., social workers, educators) are not legally entitled to ask about information on immigration status to determine eligibility for school-based services and supports. Further, even though it is legally permissible, researchers might not ask about citizenship status when conducting research because they do not want to put their participants in jeopardy or diminish trust (Reyes & Haines, 2018). Another reason why "refugee" is not used in research studies is that the term represents a heterogeneous group. Indeed, refugees come from locations around the globe; some refugees have extremely high levels of education, while others have never attended school (Bernstein & Dubois, 2018).

Notably, the term "refugee" might not be used in research because it can be perceived as deficit-based and stigmatizing. The label of "refugee" draws focus to an individual's often traumatic past, resulting in some researchers preferring to use terms like "new American" or "newcomer" in their work (Reyes & Haines, 2018). The authors of this article have conducted research focused specifically on refugee families and been told by journal reviewers to use terms "immigrant" or "culturally and linguistically diverse" in place of "refugee" in order to apply the findings to a broader context. Doing so is plausible, since the participants are also members of other groups (e.g., immigrant, students with disabilities), but it dilutes how the experiences and needs of refugee families differ from those of other populations.

Researchers engaging in research about refugee families of children with disabilities may also be sensitive to the potential marginalization and stigma involved in having a child with a disability. Indeed, appreciative research methods that enable researchers to gain participants' trust and therefore open up to them preclude asking a family to discuss difficult issues that could be perceived as deficit-based. Disability is often one of the more difficult constructs to discuss with families. The potential minoritizing caused by the labels refugee and disability also complicates recruitment; Seeking to examine a population that is marginalized based on multiple characteristics (e.g., refugee status, disability, religion) often results in difficulty recruiting participants (another phenomenon personally experienced by our authorship team).

Disability studies scholars remind us of the importance of detangling identities in order to understand the intersectionality of multiple oppressed identities (Erevelles & Minear, 2010). The importance of understanding family-professional partnerships within this group as a collective whole, knowing the heterogeneity of the group and the possible deficit-based implications, is essential to understanding phenomena affecting the families, children, and teachers in refugee resettlement sites. Not conducting research due to these limitations leads to a vacuum of research and a conglomeration of issues that are difficult to solve due to their complexity and intersectionality, thwarting innovation and evaluation of practices. The result is that, despite the desire to create the best systems and practices, educators cannot turn to research to understand how to best partner with refugee families whose children have disabilities because little research exists.

To review the landscape of research pertaining to refugee families of children with disabilities and their partnerships with professionals, we searched key scholarly databases, including Google Scholar, PsycInfo, and JStor. We limited our searches to peer-reviewed articles (including conceptual, practitioner-focused, policy-oriented, and research articles) written in English with a focus on refugees, families, and disability published during the past 20 years, from 1998 to 2018. Our initial searches resulted in articles with varying levels of relevance to the present study (e.g., Birman & Tran, 2015 study of academic engagement of Somali Bantu students in U.S. elementary schools). We further refined our search by filtering for research articles only. Then, we continued to refine the results by looking for research articles specific to refugee populations that included family-professional partnership, family engagement, or family involvement in educational or community contexts and disability. Next, we only considered articles that pertained to refugees resettled in host countries, omitting those that focused on refugees temporarily residing in countries of asylum (e.g., Sri Lanka, Kenya, Turkey). We then conducted ancestral searches on articles cited within pertinent articles.

Through this process, we identified eight peer-reviewed research articles focusing on refugees resettled in host countries whose children have disabilities and their relationship with their children's teachers. Table 1 includes synopses of these articles. While only eight research articles matched our review criteria, the findings, considered as a whole, provide important implications for the field. As stated above, the Sunshine Model provides a mechanism for systematically exploring these implications. In this section, we will use the Sunshine Model to review the implications of the accumulated body of research as related to the principles of family-professional partnership and activity type.

3.1 Principles of Family-Professional Partnerships

In this section, we utilize the principles of family-professional partnership—communication, respect, equality, competence, advocacy, commitment, and trust (Turnbull et al., 2015)—as the framework for reporting results. In the following section, we analyze the research in accordance with the partnership activities.

Communication. All eight studies included in the review emphasized the importance of communication. Some studies found that educators did not prioritize reciprocal communication with families. Haines et al. (2015a) found that communication was mostly one-way, from the school to the home. These authors found that interactions tended to be rushed, causing teachers to typically deliver information to the family without asking for family member input. In addition, teachers often read information to families during meetings, thus looking at a piece of paper instead of making eye contact, and the input the family did provide was not woven into the outcomes of the meeting. In other words, communication and goal-setting was spearheaded by the school staff, who at times solicited input from the family but did not consider this input when writing goals. Furthermore, Haines et al. (2015b) found that there was no communication with the family about their child's self-regulation and engagement skills; rather, teachers made erroneous assumptions about the family and the family's values based on the child's behavior. In addition, Miller-Gairy and Mofya (2015) found that families did not feel heard, and professionals felt that families did not participate in and were not interested in educational planning.

Even when educators prioritized communication with families, it was not always possible. Hurley et al. (2011) found that having access to timely

Table 1 Peer-Reviewed Research Articles on Family Partnership Between Refugee Families Whose Children Have Disabilities and Their Children's Teachers

Article and Overview	Key Findings	Key Implications
Beatson (2013) Seeking an understanding of how Somali Bantu refugee families perceive education and health needs of their children with disabilities, Beatson (2013) interviewed five Somali Bantu mothers and one father within a refugee community in Vermont, U.S.	• Participant-identified needs were related to access to affordable native healing ceremonies, paying for basic needs (e.g., health care, rent, disability services), knowing how to help their children with disabilities (e.g., helping with homework, dealing with challenging behavior), navigating the management of their children' behavior and special needs within the home and in public, understanding the etiology of their children's disability, and completing complex paperwork.	• Facilitate home support for families to support their children, provide homework help, and manage challenging behavior in a safe way. • Help families understand homework, behavior, and safety issues as part of IEP planning and services.
Haines et al. (2015a) Through this ethnographic case study, Haines et al. explored the partnerships between Head Start staff and a Somali refugee family whose son was under evaluation for autism spectrum disorder (ASD).	• Head Start staff offered multiple activities for family engagement that were attended by the family. • Communication was mostly one-way: from the school to the home. • The family held low expectations for partnership. • Facilitating factors included the family's willingness to participate in center activities, the family's respect for teachers, the teachers' focus on families, multiple teachers and staff members interacting with the family, and the teachers' deep caring for their students. • Impeding factors included family structure and dynamics (e.g., mother being the primary caregiver but not willing to leave children with strangers), the family's unfamiliarity with the school system and family	• Increase focus on family-professional partnerships, including more professional development and paid time allotted to meeting with families. • Bolster teachers' autonomy to flexibly meet family's needs. • Partner with resettlement agencies to ensure expectations for family partnership are part of the cultural orientations they provide.

	partnership, the Center's strict accountability measures, the numerous responsibilities and low pay for the teachers, teachers' limited knowledge of the home context, and the lack of communication among the professional team members who were working with the child and family.	• Encourage/incentivize education professionals to gather meaningful information from families. • Include refugee families in planning activities at the school or center. • Measure quality of partnership instead of solely the frequency of partnership-oriented programming.
Haines et al. (2015b) Through this ethnographic case study, the authors examined how teachers and family members of one child, Habib, from a Somali refugee family fostered his self-regulation and engagement skills in the home and at preschool.	• Adult behaviors aimed at fostering the child's skills fell into three domains: protection (ranging from restriction to freedom), intervention (ranging from low adult direction to high adult direction), and affective response (ranging from cold to warm). • Teachers' behaviors for fostering the child's skills were structured and intentional, contrasting greatly with his family's low adult direction and allowance of freedom within their apartment's protected space. • Teachers' affective responses toward Habib became warmer and their instruction even more intentional and structured while his family permitted him more freedom and recognized his good behavior more explicitly as his skills improved.	• Encourage education professionals to consider how families teach engagement and self-regulation skills to their children. • Teach families about expectations for child engagement and self-regulation in the classroom. • Explore how refugee families and school staff partner to foster children's self-regulation and engagement development.

(*Continued*)

Table 1 Peer-Reviewed Research Articles on Family Partnership Between Refugee Families Whose Children Have Disabilities and Their Children's Teachers—cont'd

Article and Overview	Key Findings	Key Implications
Hughes (2014) Through this descriptive case study, Hughes (2014) explores Tree of Life groups as a strengths-based, accessible, and nonstigmatizing alternative to traditional mental health services for children and families from refugee communities.	• An Afghani social worker was essential to getting mothers to first join the group, due to the trust they had already established. • Locating the group at a school helped wives get permission of their husbands to attend. • Mothers needed to talk and think about themselves and their own experiences before being able to work with professionals to develop positive strategies for managing their children's challenging behavior.	• Meet with refugee populations in a place that is local and familiar. • Access trusted community leaders to provide a crucial bridge to the communities served. • Host groups such as Tree of Life to (a) bring parents in contact with the school community in positive ways, (b) reach children and families from refugee communities who might not otherwise access traditional mental health services, and (c) integrate cultural understandings and norms into therapeutic work so that participants find their own way forward that fits with their culture and individual perspectives.

Hurley et al. (2011) Hurley et al. interviewed 25 early childhood educators to explore their experiences working with preschool children and their families who are members of a small New England refugee resettlement community.	• Participants cited challenges and facilitators related to communication, including (a) lack of access to timely, cost effective, and accurate interpretation services, which resulted in inadequate communication with families, and (b) mismatch in the language of the teacher and the refugee child contributed to "emotional upset" on the part of the child in the classroom. • Communication was enhanced by the use of sign language, pictures, facial expressions, and affection. • Participants cited cultural complexity challenges, including the teachers' lack of cultural competence, cultural differences in information sharing, and cultural differences around child safety and rules. • Participants identified the benefits of accessing cultural liaisons who were members of the refugee community to help facilitate communication and partnership.	• Enhance professional development related to cultural competence for teachers working within refugee resettlement cities. • Facilitate timely, accurate, and cost-effective interpreter services for educators and families • Facilitate educators access to cultural liaisons who are members of the same refugee resettlement communities as students/families. • Investigate research-based communication strategies teachers can use to bridge languages with students to help offset the behavioral challenges that may arise when young children are not able to communicate directly with teachers and peers.

(Continued)

Table 1 Peer-Reviewed Research Articles on Family Partnership Between Refugee Families Whose Children Have Disabilities and Their Children's Teachers—cont'd

Article and Overview	Key Findings	Key Implications
Hurley et al. (2014) Through interviews with 28 preschool service providers, Hurley et al. sought to highlight their perspectives on challenges and practices implemented when working with refugee families whose preschool aged children had disabilities.	• Conflicts exist amongst preschool service providers around how quickly a child should be evaluated for special education, with early childhood educators wanting special education teams to react more quickly while early childhood special educators were faced with limited valid assessment tools and the difficulty of administering evaluations when children do not speak English and have not spent time outside of the home. • Service providers noted that parents are not proactive in pursuing services for their children with disabilities due to a desire to assimilate, being afraid to ask for services, their own post-traumatic stress, and their perceptions of their child's disability diagnosis not being a priority based on their experiences. • Participants noted cultural dissonance with families who did not want their child evaluated due to the meetings, paperwork, and differing priorities. • Service providers described helpful practices in partnering with families to determine whether the child has a disability, including observing children in play and comparing their development to their siblings and asking families about the child's language development in their native languages. • Refugee children are not receiving evaluations for special education in the same timely manner as preschoolers with suspected delays from other cultural groups.	• Develop standardized assessments and evidence based practices for assessing refugee children. • Develop strategies educators can use to help refugee families participate in their children's educational programming and understand the evaluation process. • Recruit more diverse teacher candidates in universities, including refugees and immigrants. • Create evidence-based practices for partnering with families in the evaluation process and for serving families and children who are refugees.

Hurley et al. (2017) Through qualitative interviews with nine multicultural liaisons who worked for two school districts in a New England refugee resettlement city, the authors sought to identify indicators that IEP teams should consider when preparing for and conducting IEP meetings with recently resettled refugee families of children with disabilities.	• Teachers must understand the difference between immigrants and refugees, learn about families' cultures and be sensitive to cultural differences, understand how families view their roles and the teachers' roles in their child's education, and seek to understand how disability is perceived in their culture. • Teachers should prepare families and cultural liaisons for the IEP meeting, making sure the purpose of the meeting is clear, all forms and rights are translated and given to the families in advance of the meeting, and all documents are reviewed in advance with the cultural liaison/interpreter. • Teachers should provide food and drinks at the IEP meeting to help create a more relaxed environment. • Long meetings should be avoided as they can result in loss of focus or the tendency to "rush." An alternative to long meetings would to schedule multiple meetings that are shorter in duration. • During meetings, teachers should talk slowly, use short statements and simple words; avoid acronyms and idioms; make eye contact with the family (not the cultural liaison); and listen to the family without interruption. • In order to facilitate partnership with refugee families, educators need to demonstrate compassion and respect during IEP meetings.	• Provide teachers access to professional development related to cultural competence and sensitivity specific to the refugee populations in their community, classroom, and school. • Facilitate teacher skills in communicating with families while using an interpreter, and they should learn how to be sensitive in their communication strategies specific to various cultures. • Engage IEP team members in more significant advanced planning when they involve cultural liaisons and refugee families. • Embed relationship-building strategies grounded in compassion and respect within IEP meetings.

(Continued)

Table 1 Peer-Reviewed Research Articles on Family Partnership Between Refugee Families Whose Children Have Disabilities and Their Children's Teachers—cont'd

Article and Overview	Key Findings	Key Implications
Miller-Gairy and Mofya (2015) Through an ethnographic study involving focus groups, observations, and interviews, Miller-Gairy and Mofya examined both how culture and tradition shape perceptions and expectations of Somali mothers of children with autism and how service providers experience working with such families.	• Mothers' perceptions of autism were that it was a U.S.-centric disease that their child would not have gotten if they had stayed in Somalia. • Mothers felt they were rarely given the opportunity to speak with the therapist because they were foreign. • Gender as it relates to cultural norms was also an issue for both parents and providers (i.e., mothers had problems working with men, providers did not understand cultural norms of fathers not being involved). • Mothers felt alienated during IEP meetings and felt that professionals stated an endless list of problems instead of listening to their concerns. • Mothers did not feel welcome at the school and did not trust educators. • Providers identified basic communication barriers, including needing children to translate for families and mothers showing up to therapy sessions with many kids. • Providers noted that parents failed to engage in conversation with them and follow through with recommendations or referrals.	• Improve communication between stakeholders. • Facilitate provider understanding of basic cultural norms (e.g., gender roles, African concept of family). • Establish trusting relationships in order for partnership to come to fruition.

interpretation services was a barrier for communicating with refugee families. One participant stated that "by the time you get [an interpreter], the issue is over" (p. 162). Additionally, Hurley et al. (2017) underscored the importance of families understanding the purpose of the Individualized Education Program (IEP) meeting and knowing their rights before arriving for the meeting. These authors urged educators to meet with cultural liaisons, or school personnel who are part of the refugee communities but who speak their native language as well as English fluently and can help interpret cultural issues as well as language, before the IEP meeting to go through all the processes and jargon to ensure that communication was as accurate and clear as possible. Furthermore, Hurley et al. (2017) suggested that educators use simple words, short statements, and pause often for cultural liaisons to interpret for families. They also underscored the importance of educators making eye contact and talking directly to families, not the cultural liaison. Similarly, Beatson (2013) found that clear communication was absolutely requisite for partnering with Somali Bantu families. This author expressed that etiology needed to be repeated until understood, and, like Hurley, Warren, Habalow, Weber, and Tousignant (2014, 2017), interpreters were important for making sure this information was culturally-situated and understood.

Respect. Many studies found that educators did not show respect to the families of their students. For example, Hurley et al. (2017) found that cultural liaisons saw teachers treat families with a lack of respect. One participant from this study stated that "if you don't know the language, people treat you like you not halfway human which is hurting" (p. 41). Another participant suggested that teachers should take a class on "having a heart ... [Teachers] belong to a social class where they have a certain job and they don't even know they're acting like this" (p. 41). In another study, Hurley et al. (2011) found that educators had an awareness that some of the school policies are not respectful of other cultures (e.g., policies related to privacy and safety), and they expressed concern that these policies affected their ability to build relationships with families. Participants "expressed discomfort about imposing their culture's standards concerning child safety onto the refugee families" (p. 163). However, the educators did not know how to change policies or practices that they believed were not respectful of other cultures. Haines et al. (2015a) found that the rushed interactions between educators and the family, due to strict accountability measures for conferences, limited teachers' showing of respect.

On the other hand, some studies highlighted respectful interactions between professionals and families. Participants expressed respect for families through the strengths-based, culturally-competent Tree of Life activity described by Hughes (2014). The Tree of Life activity uses the tree as a metaphor and enables families to share stories about their lives that are woven into solutions to their self-identified problems. Beatson (2013) also explained that understanding the families' preferred methods for raising their children with disabilities enables practitioners to respect those techniques while potentially building on them with professional expertise.

Professional competence. Few articles directly discussed the importance of professional competence. Haines et al. (2015a,b) found that the family deferred to their child's teachers and trusted them due to their status as teachers and also because they saw the genuine care teachers had for their child. Hurley et al. (2014, 2017) found that educators needed to increase their knowledge and skills related to cultural responsiveness and showing compassion and respect to refugee families.

Commitment. Several articles discussed the need for educators to be committed to refugee families because partnering with these families can be more complex than partnering with other families. Beatson (2013) stated that practitioners should meet families in their homes. Hughes (2014) found that using the Tree of Life process required an extensive, but worthwhile, time commitment. Hurley et al. (2011) found that teachers showed their commitment to refugee children and families by trying different communication methods and hiring cultural liaisons. Hurley et al. (2017) also identified the need for educators to go above and beyond their typical duties by working with cultural liaisons to understand the IEP process and jargon as well as translate all documents. These authors also called for providing food during meetings, which can also demonstrate commitment.

Equality. Two studies explicitly highlighted the lack of equality in the relationships between family and professionals, though all studies alluded to inequality. For example, teachers in Hurley et al. (2011) study articulated that their lack of access to quality and timely interpreters resulted in inequality in communication with refugee families. One participant from this study stated, "We never had a parent-teacher conference this year with either of our [refugee] children because we couldn't set up times with the interpreters … the other [English-speaking] parents we talk to about every day" (p. 162). In addition, Hurley et al. (2017) identified numerous implications for ensuring equality, including making sure all information is shared in understandable ways.

Advocacy. None of the eight studies we reviewed explicitly addressed the principle of advocacy in research findings.

Trust. The central tenet of family-professional partnerships is trust. Many studies discussed the importance of trust. Hughes (2014) found that the link to community members was absolutely essential for garnering trust with families involved in the Tree of Life person-centered planning process. This author emphasized the necessity of building trust with families before discussing any problems or deficits with them. Hurley et al. (2011) identified teachers' lack of cultural competence as impeding trust. For example, one participant explained that a parent was horrified when the teacher sent home a picture of the child petting a service dog at school. In the child's culture, dogs were seen as disgusting and unsafe, and the family was dismayed that the teacher let the child touch the dog. In addition, these authors identified that the educator's lack of direct communication with the students and families was a barrier to trust. Miller-Gairy and Mofya (2015) also identified the lack of trust as a major barrier to partnership between Somali Bantu mothers and their children's teachers.

3.2 Partnership Activities

The Sunshine Model also identifies the "what" of partnership, or the activities that families and professionals do together through partnership. These partnership activities include determining and meeting needs; obtaining services and supports; monitoring services and supports; connecting home, school, and community; and advocating for systems improvement (Haines et al., 2017). We organize the findings presented in the eight articles included in this review according to these partnership activities.

Determining and meeting needs. Several articles discussed determining and meeting needs. Haines et al. (2015a) found that Head Start policy required educators to seek family input on determining child needs, but that, in practice, family input was not included. Instead, the policy did not translate to practice due to rushed conferences and a focus on getting the task done (i.e., checking it off the requisite checklist) without fulfilling the purpose of the task (i.e., seeking meaningful family input). In addition, Haines et al. (2015b) found that teachers evaluated the child for autism due to his lack of self-regulation and engagement skills. The teachers neither sought understanding of the child's self-regulation and engagement skills as manifested or fostered in the home nor discussed the child's behavior at the center with his family before referring him for special education diagnosis. If they had sought this information, they would have learned that the family's child-rearing practices emphasized freedom within a safe environment and did not foster these skills in the same way as the pedagogical techniques of the center.

Some studies identified promising techniques for determining and meeting needs. Hughes (2014) found that the Tree of Life process was successful at helping families and social workers determine child needs openly and through partnership. In a similar vein, Hurley et al. (2014) found that child needs should be determined through discussions with families in which families compare children's development to their siblings,' asking the family about the child's use of the native language(s), and observing the child playing in their natural environment. Miller-Gairy and Mofya (2015) found that only four of the nine children with autism received services and supports because the mothers of the other five did not believe they needed them; this demonstrates that they were part of the decision-making process for determining needs.

Obtaining services and supports. While Haines et al. (2015a,b) found that the family did not know their son was being evaluated for special education even though they signed the consent for evaluation, other studies highlighted effective techniques for obtaining services and supports. Beatson (2013) found that practitioners should ask families what they need. In addition, practitioners should be flexible with the approaches they use and always make sure families understand approaches and are comfortable with them. Hughes (2014) employed a strength-based narrative methodology, using the tree as a creative metaphor, thus enabling refugee mothers to develop empowering stories about their lives which were rooted in their cultural and social histories. From this secure base, mothers were able to develop shared, culturally appropriate solutions to their problems, rather than being forced into a Western mode of traditional mental health supports.

Monitoring Services and Supports. Other than Miller-Gairy and Mofya's (2015) finding that IEP meetings were not pleasant experiences for the mothers who participated in their study because they felt unheard, unwelcome, and disrespected, no study focused on monitoring services and supports.

Connecting home, school, and community. Hughes (2014) argued that the Tree of Life process is a great way to bring together family, school, and community in a positive, strengths-based way. All other studies reviewed highlighted the missed opportunity to bring together the family, school, and community.

4. IMPLICATIONS

The research reviewed in this manuscript offers interrelated implications that reflect the principles of family-professional partnerships and partnership activities outlined in the Sunshine Model (see Fig. 1). Numerous studies including those conducted by Hughes (2014), Hurley et al. (2011; 2017), and Miller-Gairy and Mofya (2015) called for greater communication between families and professionals characterized by trust, respect, and equality. These implications emphasized the importance of access to interpreters and cultural liaisons, adherence to cultural norms, and building trust by meeting in a place a refugee family member feels comfortable among people with whom they have existing, trusting relationships. Research also provided implications related to the principle of professional competence by calling for professional development for partnering with refugee families, including understanding how various cultures and refugee experiences interact with commonly-held Western values and customs and reconciling cultural differences related to expectations for skills such as self-regulation, behavior, and homework (Beatson, 2013; Haines et al., 2015a,b; Hughes, 2014; Hurley et al., 2014, 2017). Haines et al. (2015a) also described implications related to professional competence to determine and meet needs, including supporting teacher autonomy. Related to the partnership principle of commitment, these authors also suggest that educators receive paid time to meet with families.

Other implications, such as professionals partnering with resettlement agencies (Haines et al., 2015a); developing standardized, evidence-based instruments for assessing refugee students (Hurley et al., 2014); and meaningfully including refugee families in school and student educational planning (Beatson, 2013; Haines et al., 2015a,b; Hurley et al., 2014, 2017) reflect the partnership principles of equality, competence, and commitment and the partnership activities of connecting home, school, and community; determining and meeting needs; and monitoring services and supports. Further, implications related to recruiting more diverse teacher candidates, including refugees and other immigrants, offered by Hurley et al. (2014) have potential implications for all partnership principles and activities.

Many findings of this literature review specific to refugee populations align with research related to the broader culturally and linguistically diverse community. Within the need for open communication amongst families and professionals, there are numerous commonalities. For example, research documents the importance of interpreters in facilitating communication with Spanish-speaking families (e.g., Francis et al., 2018; Hughes, Valle-Riestra, & Arguelles, 2008; Pang, 2011; Salas, 2004). In addition, educational research indicates a need for professional development (Gothberg et al., 2018) and effective interagency collaboration (Francis et al., 2018) to better partner with and support culturally and linguistically diverse families. Hurley et al. (2017) recommended employing cultural liaisons to assist in communication with diverse families, which aligns with previous research using promotoras, or Latino community workers, to assist families in changing their approaches with children with IDD (Magana, Lopez, Paradiso de Sayu, & Miranda, 2014).

Research clearly documents the importance of advocacy on behalf of culturally and linguistically diverse families (Burke & Goldman, 2018). Given that marginalized families face greater barriers in accessing services for their children with disabilities (Gothberg et al., 2018), and refugee families may not fully understand the plethora of services available to meet their children's needs nor their children's right to access them when appropriate, advocacy is an especially necessary partnership principle for the refugee population. There are currently no advocacy trainings or advocacy research specifically among refugee families, however, and this is a significant gap.

Advocacy and leadership training for refugee families could also help provide a healthy dose of skepticism for families, which is in part the checks and balances system established by the parent participation principle of IDEA. Lea (2006) found that early interventionists demonstrated their respect for and gained the respect of the African-American teenage mother participants through developing strong relationships and getting to know them as individuals. The skepticism discovered by Lea, though so strong that it was a barrier to partnership, could actually help ensure that services and supports are appropriate and relevant to families' lives. Indeed, as expressed in Miller-Gairy and Mofya's (2015) research, trust might not exist due to inappropriate interactions and a lack of cultural responsiveness, but healthy ways of communicating and working together despite violations of trust would benefit family, child, and teacher. Other studies specific to refugees, however, found that some families have a deference to professionals without first developing these relationships, due at least in part to the attitude that the teacher knows what is best for the student as well as the families' limited knowledge of American school systems and pedagogies (Haines et al., 2015a). Such one-sided educational planning enables educators to ignore family perspectives, wisdom, and systems, and perpetuates the idea that the teacher knows what is best for the child and family. The family is ultimately responsible for the child throughout the lifespan; reinforcing such hierarchical and narrow views of education and service-provision could end up muting family and student voice.

Research on family-professional partnerships for refugee families of children with disabilities is extremely limited and, even though much of the research conducted on family partnerships with families whose children have disabilities and other historically marginalized identities might pertain to this population, there is a need to improve the research base on this specific (and heterogenous) population due to the compounding nature of the multiple potential barriers to forming successful partnerships with them. Refugees are underrepresented in special education research, as are English learners. In fact, Sinclair et al. (2018), in their examination of intervention studies in 12 peer-reviewed special education journals from 2000–16, noted that only 3.2% of the 495 included articles reported participants who were English language learners. We contend that refugee resettlement communities deserve access to research-based strategies that will help educators partner with families to meet the needs of students with disabilities. To meet this need, future research should examine the complexity of developing positive family-professional partnership practices for refugee families of children with disabilities. In order to do this, the field should not discourage the term "refugee" as a descriptor of participants. Although refugees are a heterogenous group, educators working with refugee families and children need to be able to turn to a research base to guide their practice. Lumping research focused on refugees with research focused on the broader immigrant population washes out the specific nuances of working with the refugee population. Research questions should build on the findings of this review and explore effective techniques to foster family-professional partnerships as well as common barriers and solutions to creating these relationships. Research should also highlight successful existing and emerging/experimental practices facilitating family-professional partnerships in education and other fields (e.g., medicine, social services) through a variety of methods. For example, in-depth case studies across various refugee populations, student age groups, and disability types should be included in research agendas as this method offers rich, contextual information that professionals need in order to learn about and adopt partnership practices with refugee families. Student voice was also notably absent in the studies we reviewed, warranting future research exploring student perceptions and experiences of family-professional partnerships. It is imperative that this research include cultural insiders and cultural liaisons in order to obtain access and meaningful and candid information from families (Reyes & Haines, 2018).

As indicated in the previous section, two areas with less research than others are the partnership principle of advocacy and the partnership activity of monitoring services and supports. It is imperative that educators advocate for the refugee families with whom they work in partnership by taking the time to get to know the families and their concerns for their children. Special educators are in a great position to advocate for the families with whom they partner, and these advocacy efforts should also be highlighted through research. In addition, teacher preparation programs can bolster their graduates' understanding of the role of advocacy by emphasizing culturally responsive practice and including in their classes service-learning components involving getting to know refugee families. Similarly, professional development programs could focus on informing educators about local refugee populations and invite community leaders to share information and strategies to partner with families. It is important for refugee families to learn to become advocates and leaders, and future research should investigate advocacy trainings within the refugee community.

It is also critical that families and professionals partner in monitoring services and supports. This may be accomplished through dedicated funding allocations for interpreters and cultural liaisons as well as potential changes to educational and resettlement policies that reflect interagency collaboration, similar to those outlined in the Workforce Innovation and Opportunity Act (2014). Paired with increasing advocacy efforts, refugee families should be involved in determining what services and supports work for their children with disabilities and their family. Having an advocacy voice and participating in monitoring services and supports could help hold service providers to a higher level of accountability while also augmenting refugee family engagement in their children's education.

5. CONCLUSION

In this article, we responded to a need to synthesize research related to family-professional partnerships with refugee families whose children have disabilities. The expectation of family-professional partnerships in the U.S. educational system, especially when the children have disabilities or struggle in school, is extremely important but yet often remains implied rather than made explicit for refugee families. Our goal for this article was to portray the research base related to family-professional partnerships for refugee families of children with disabilities and who are resettled in host countries. We defined "refugee" and provided background on refugee populations living in the U.S. We also discussed why the topic of family-professional partnerships is important, especially for refugee populations. After outlining the Sunshine Model (Haines et al., 2017), we discussed the existing research on family-professional partnerships with refugee families of children with disabilities in host countries of resettlement. Finally, we called for increased attention to family-professional partnerships with refugee families whose children have disabilities. Improving family-professional partnerships for refugee families whose children have disabilities is a matter of social justice, and we hope this review serves as a call to increase this line of research and strengthen these practices.

ACKNOWLEDGMENT

This research was supported by the Center for Disability and Community Inclusion at the University of Vermont.

REFERENCES

Aldersey, H. M., & Haines, S. J. (2017). Teaching students with intellectual disabilities in Kinshasa, democratic Republic of Congo. *Journal of International Special Needs Education, 20*(2), 90–100.

Atwell, R., Gifford, S., & McDonald-Wilmsen, B. (2009). Resettled refugee families and their Children's Futures: Coherence, hope and support. *Journal of Comparative Family Studies, 40*(5), 677–697. Retrieved from: http://www.jstor.org/stable/41604320.

Beatson, J. E. (2013). Supporting Somali Bantu mothers of children with disabilities. *Pediatric Nursing, 39*(3), 142–145.

Bernstein, H., & Dubois, N. (April 2018). *Bringing evidence to the refugee integration debate.* Retrieved from the Urban Institute website: https://www.urban.org/sites/default/files/publication/97771/bringing_evidence_to_the_refugee_integration_debate_0.pdf.

Birman, D., & Tran, N. (2015). *The academic engagement of newly arriving Somali Bantu students in a U. S. elementary school.* Washington, DC: Migration Policy Institute. Retrieved from: www.migrationpolicy.org/research/acedmic-engagement-newly-arriving-somali-bantu-students-us-elementary-school.

Birman, D., Trickett, E. J., & Bacchus, N. (2001). *Somali youth report.* The Maryland Office for New Americans. Retrieved from: http://www.springinstitute.org/Files/marylandreport.pdfBlue.

Blackwell, W. H., & Rossetti, Z. S. (2014). The development of individualized education programs: Where have we been and where should we go now? *Sage Open, 4*(2), 2158244014530411.

Blue-Banning, M., Summers, J. A., Frankland, H. C., Nelson, L. L., & Beegle, G. (2004). Dimensions of family and professional partnerships: Constructive guidelines for collaboration. *Exceptional Children, 70*, 167–184.

Bryan, J., & Henry, L. (2012). A model for building school-family-community partnerships: Principles and process. *Journal of Counseling and Development, 90*, 408–420. https://doi.org/10.1002/j.1556-6676.2012.00052.x.

Burke, M., & Goldman, S. (2018). Special education advocacy among culturally and linguistically diverse families. *Journal of Research in Special Educational Needs.* https://doi.org/10.111/1471-3802.12413.

Burke, M., & Hodapp, R. (2014). Relating stress of mothers of children with developmental disabilities to family-school partnerships. *Intellectual and Developmental Disabilities, 52*, 13–23.

Cooper, C. W., Riehl, C. J., & Hasan, A. L. (2010). Leading and learning with diverse families in schools: Critical epistemology amid communities of practice. *Journal of School Leadership, 20*, 758–788. Retrieved from: https://eric.ed.gov/?id=EJ916124.

Dachyshyn, D., & Kirova, A. (2008). Understanding childhoods in-between: Sudanese refugee and children's transition from home to preschool. Theme issue on Early Childhood Education and Care. *Research in Comparative and International Education, 3*(3), 281–294.

Dávila, B. (2015). Critical race theory, disability microaggressions and Latina/o student experiences in special education. *Race, Ethnicity and Education, 18*, 443–468. https://doi.org/10.1080/13613324.2014.885422.

Epstein, J. L., & Sanders, M. G. (2006). Prospects for change: Preparing educators for school, family, and community partnerships. *Peabody Journal of Education, 81*(2), 81–120. https://doi.org/10.1207/S15327930pje8102_5.

Erevelles, N., & Minear, A. (2010). Unspeakable offenses: Untangling race and disability in discourses of intersectionality. *Journal of Literary & Cultural Disability Studies, 4*(2), 127–146. https://doi.org/10.3828/jlcds.2010.11.

Eskow, K. G., Summers, J. A., Chasson, G. S., & Mitchell, R. (2018). The association between family-teacher partnership satisfaction and outcomes of academic progress and quality of life for children/youth with autism. *Journal of Policy and Practice in Intellectual Disabilities*. https://doi.org/10.1111/jppi.12221.

Every student succeeds Act of 2015, pub. L. No. 114-95 § 114 stat. 1177.(2015-2016).

Ferguson, D. L. (2008). International trends in inclusive education: The continuing challenge to teach each one and everyone. *European Journal of Special Needs Education, 23*(2), 109–120. https://doi.org/10.1080/08856250801946236.

Foley, K. R., Blackmore, A. M., Girdler, S., O'Donnell, M., Glauert, R., Llewellyn, G., & Leonard, H. (2012). *To feel belonged:* The voices of children and youth with disabilities on the meaning of wellbeing. *Child Indicators Research, 5*, 375–391. https://doi.org/10.1007/s12187-011-9134-2.

Francis, G. L., Blue-Banning, M., Haines, S. J., Turnbull, A. P., & Gross, J. M. S. (2016). Building "our school:" Parental perspectives for building trusting family-professional partnerships. *Preventing School Failure, 60*, 329–336. https://doi.org/10.1080/1045988X.2016.1164115.

Francis, G. L., Gross, J. M. S., Lavin, C., Casarez, L., & Sheets, N. (2018). *Hispanic caregiver's experiences supporting positive post-school outcomes for young adults with disabilities*. Manuscript accepted *to Intellectual and Developmental Disabilities* (Still in press).

Francis, G. L., Haines, S. J., & Nagro, S. (2017). Developing relationships with immigrant families: Learning by asking the right questions. *Teaching Exceptional Children*. https://doi.org/10.1177/0040059917720778.

Francis, G. L., Mueller, T. G., & Turnbull, H. R. (2018). *Social role valorization of caregivers in school systems: The influence of terminology in federal education legislation*. Manuscript under review.

Giovacco-Johnson, T. (2009). Portraits of partnership: The hopes and dreams project. *Early Childhood Education Journal, 37*(2), 127–135.

Goddard, R. D., Tschannen-Moran, M., & Hoy, W. K. (2001). A multilevel examination of the distribution and effects of teacher trust in students and parents in urban elementary schools. *The Elementary School Journal, 102*(1), 3–17.

Gothberg, J. E., Greene, G., & Kohler, P. D. (2018). District implementation of research-based practices for transition planning with culturally and linguistically diverse youth with disabilities and their families. *Career Development and Transition for Exceptional Individuals*. https://doi.org/10.1177/2165143418762794.

Haines, S. J., & Francis, G. L. (April 2016). Family partnership with refugee families in the us whose children have disabilities: A review of the literature. In *Poster presented at the annual meeting of the council for exceptional children, St. Louis, MO*.

Haines, S. J., & Reyes, C. (April 2018). Examining the complexity of family-professional partnerships between refugee families and their children's teachers. In *Paper presented at the annual meeting of the American educational research association, New York city, NY*.

Haines, S. J., McCart, A., & Turnbull, A. P. (2013). Family engagement within early childhood Response to Intervention. In V. Buysse, & E. Peisner-Feinberg (Eds.), *Handbook on response to intervention (RTI) in early childhood* (pp. 313–324). New York: Paul H. Brookes.

Haines, S. J., Summers, J. A., Turnbull, A. P., & Turnbull, H. R. (2015a). Family partnership with a Head Start agency: A case study of a refugee family, National Head Start Research Association's Dialog. *17*(4), 22–49. https://journals.uncc.edu/dialog/article/view/168/354.

Haines, S. J., Summers, J. A., Turnbull, A. P., Palmer, S. B., & Turnbull, H. R. (2015b). Fostering Habib's engagement and self-regulation: A case study of a child from a refugee family at home and preschool. *Topics in Early Childhood Special Education, 35*(1), 28–39. https://doi.org/10.1177/0271121414552905.

Haines, S. J., Francis, G. L., Mueller, T., Chiu, C. Y., Burke, M., Holdren, N., ... Turnbull, A. P. (2017). Reconceptualizing family-professional partnership for inclusive schools: A call to action. *Inclusion, 5*(4), 234–247. https://doi.org/10.1352/2326-6988-5.4.234.

Harry, B. H. (2008). Collaboration with culturally and linguistically diverse families: Ideal versus reality. *Exceptional Children, 51*, 327–388. https://doi.org/10.1177/001440290807400306.

He, Y., Bettez, S. C., & Levin, B. B. (2017). Imagined community of education: Voices from refugees and immigrants. *Urban Education, 52*, 957–985.

Henderson, A. T., & Mapp, K. L. (2002). *A new wave of evidence: The impact of school, family and community connections on student achievement*. Austin, TX: Southwest Educational Development.

Hill, N. E., & Taylor, L. C. (2004). Parental school involvement and children's academic achievement: Pragmatics and issues. *Current Directions in Psychological Science, 13*(4), 161–164. https://doi.org/10.1111/j.0963-72141.2004.00298.x.

Hoy, W. (2012). School characteristics that make a difference for the achievement of all students: A 40-year odyssey. *Journal of Educational Administration, 50*(1), 76–97. https://doi.org/10.1108/09578231211196078.

Hughes, G. (2014). Finding a voice through 'the tree of life': A strength based approach to mental health for refugee children and families in schools. *Clinical Child Psychology and Psychiatry, 19*(1), 139–153.

Hughes, M. T., Valle-Riestra, D. M., & Arguelles, M. E. (2008). The voices of Latino families raising children with special needs. *Journal of Latinos and Education, 7*(3), 241–257. https://doi.org/10.1080/15348430802100337.

Hurley, J. J., Clark, D. W., Fonseca-Foster, K. A., Pyne, S. K., & Warren, R. A. (2017). Collaboration during IEP and IFSP meetings in a refugee resettlement community: Lessons from cultural liaisons. *Multiple Voices for Ethnically Diverse Exceptional Learners, 17*(2), 34–44.

Hurley, J. J., Medici, A., Stewart, E., & Cohen, Z. (2011). Supporting preschoolers and their families who are recently resettled refugees. *Multicultural Perspectives, 13*(3), 160–166. https://doi.org/10.1080/15210960.2011.594400.

Hurley, J. J., Saini, S., Warren, R. A., & Carberry, A. J. (2013). Use of the pyramid model for supporting preschool refugees. *Early Child Development and Care, 183*(1), 75–91.

Hurley, J. J., Warren, R. A., Habalow, R. D., Weber, L. E., & Tousignant, S. R. (2014). Early childhood special education in a refugee resettlement community: Challenges and innovative practices. *Early Child Development and Care, 184*, 50–62. https://doi.org/10.1080/03004430.2013.769214.

Hwa-Froelich, D. A., & Westby, C. E. (2003). Frameworks of education: Perspectives of southeast Asian parents and Head Start staff. *Language, Speech, and Hearing Services in Schools, 34*, 299–319.

Individuals with disabilities education Act, 20 U.S.C. § 1400.(2004).

Isik-Ercan, Z. (2012). In pursuit of a new perspective in the education of children of the refugees: Advocacy for the "family". *Educational Sciences: Theory and Practice, 12*, 3025–3038. https://doi.org/10.1111/1475-3588.00286.

Jegatheesan, B. (2009). Cross-cultural issues in parent-professional interactions: A qualitative study of perceptions of Asian American mothers of children with developmental disabilities. *Research and Practice for Persons with Severe Disabilities, 34*, 123–136.

Kalyanpur, M., & Harry, B. (2012). *Cultural reciprocity in special education: Building family-professional relationships*. Baltimore, MD: Paul H. Brooks.

Kyzar, K. B., Brady, S., Summers, J. A., Haines, S. J., & Turnbull, A. P. (2016). Services and supports, partnership, and family quality of life: Focus on deaf-blindness. *Exceptional Children, 83*(1), 77–91. https://doi.org/10.1177/0014402916655432.

Kyzar, K., Mueller, T. G., Francis, G. L., & Haines, S. J. (February 2018). Examining the state of special education training opportunities for family-professional partnership practices. In *Paper presented at the annual meeting of council for exceptional children, Tampa, FL.*

Landmark, L. J., Roberts, E. L., & Zhang, D. (2013). Educators' beliefs and practices about parent involvement in transition planning. *Career Development and Transition for Exceptional Individuals, 36*, 114–123. https://doi.org/10.1177/2165143412463047.

LaRocque, M., Kleiman, I., & Darling, S. M. (2011). Parental involvement: The missing link in school achievement. *Preventing School Failure, 55*(3), 115–122. https://doi.org/10.1080/10459880903472876.

Lawson, N. L. (2003). Pursuing and securing collaboration to improve results. In M. Brabeck, M. Walsh, & R. Latta (Eds.), Meeting at the hyphen, *102nd yearbook of the national society for the study of education, Part II* (pp. 45–71). Chicago: University of Chicago Press.

Lea, D. (2006). 'You don't know me *like that*': Patterns of disconnect between adolescent mothers of children with disabilities and their early interventionists. *Journal of Early Intervention, 28*, 264–282.

Leonard, J. (2011). Using Brofenbrenner's ecological theory to understand community partnerships: A historical case study of one urban high school. *Urban Education, 46*, 987–1010. https://doi.org/10.1177/0042085911400337.

Lo, L. (2012). Demystifying the IEP process for diverse parents of children with disabilities. *Teaching Exceptional Children, 44*, 14–20. https://doi.org/10.1177/004005991204400302.

Magana, S., Lopez, K., Paradiso de Sayu, R., & Miranda, E. (2014). Chapter two- Use of promotoras de salud in interventions with Latino families of children with IDD. *International Review of Research in Developmental Disabilities, 47*, 39–75. https://doi.org/10.1016/B978-0-12-800278-0.00002-6.

Mandic, C. M., Rudd, R., Hedir, T., & Acevedo-Garcia, D. (2012). Readability of special education procedural safeguards. *The Journal of Special Education, 45*, 195–203. https://doi.org/10.1177/0022466910362774.

Mapp, K., & Hong, S. (2010). Debunking the myth of the hard-to-reach parent. In S. L. Christenen, & A. L. Reschly (Eds.), *Handbook of school-family partnerships* (pp. 345–361). New York, NY: Routledge.

Markow, D., Macia, L., & Lee, H. (2013). *The MetLife survey of the American teacher: Challenges for school leadership*. New York, NY: Metropolitan Life Insurance Company.

McBrien, J. L. (2005). Educational needs and barriers for refugee students in the United States: A review of the literature. *Review of Educational Research, 75*(3), 329–364. https://doi.org/10.3102/00346543075003329.

McBrien, J. L. (2011). The importance of context: Vietnamese, Somali, and Iranian refugee mothers discuss their resettled lives and involvement in their children's education. *Compare: A Journal of Comparative and International Education, 41*, 75–90.

Miller-Gairy, S., & Mofya, S. (2015). Elements of culture and tradition that shape the perceptions and expectations of Somali refugee mothers about autism spectrum disorder. *International Journal of Child and Adolescent Health, 8*(4), 425–438.

Minhas, R. S. (2014). The double disability of refugee children. *Academic Pediatrics, 2014*(1), 8–9. https://doi.org/10.1016/j.acap.2013.11.004.

Pang, Y. (2011). Barriers and solutions in involving culturally and linguistically diverse families in the IFSP/IEP process. *Making Connections: Interdisciplinary Approaches to Cultural Diversity, 12*(2), 42–51.

Perry, K. H. (2009). Genres, contexts, and literacy practices: Literacy brokering among Sudanese refugee families. *Reading Research Quarterly, 44*(3), 25–276.

Phillips, E. (2008). When parents aren't enough: External advocacy in special education. *The Yale Law Journal, 117*(8), 1804–1852.

Plyer v. Doe, 457 U. S. 202.(1982).

Reyes, C., & Haines, S. J. (April 2018). Examining the ethics and humanizing approaches of conducting research with families with refugee experience. In *Paper presented at the annual meeting of the American education research Association. New York, NY. PR.*

Salas, L. (2004). Individualized educational plan (IEP) meetings and Mexican American parents: Let's talk about it. *Journal of Latinos and Education, 3*(3), 181–192.

Schiller, N., Boggis, J., Messenger, M., & Douglas, M. (2009). *Refugee resettlement in New Hampshire: Pathways and barriers to building community*. Durham: University of New Hampshire.

Sinclair, J., Hansen, S. G., Machalicek, W., Knowles, C., Hirana, K., Dolata, A. W., … Murray, C. (2018). A 16-year review of participant diversity in intervention research across a selection of 12 special education journals. *Exceptional Children, 84*(3), 312–329. https://doi.org/10.1177/0014402918756989.

Skrtic, T. M., Sailor, W., & Gee, K. (1996). Voice, collaboration, and Inclusion: Democratic themes in educational and social reform initiatives. *Remedial and Special Education, 17*, 142–157.

Tadesse, S. (2014). Parent involvement: Perceived encouragement and barriers to African refugee parent and teacher relationships. *Childhood Education, 90*, 298–305. https://doi.org/10.1080/00094056.2014.937275.

Tadesse, S., Hoot, J., & Watson-Thompson, O. (2009). Exploring the special needs of African refugee children in U.S. schools. *Childhood Education, 85*(6), 352–356.

Tonelson, S. W., & Waters, R. (1993). Interagency collaboration. In B. Billingsly (Ed.), *Program leadership in special education* (pp. 55–66). Richmond, VA: Virginia Department of Education.

Tryer, R. A., & Fazel, M. (2014). School and community-based interventions for refugee and asylum seeking children: A systematic review. *PLoS One, 9*(2), e89359. https://doi.org/10.1371/journal.pone.0089359.

Tschannen-Moran, M. (2014). *Trust matters: Leadership for successful schools*. San Francisco, CA: Jossey-Bass.

Turnbull, H. R., Stowe, M., & Huerta, N. (2007). *Free appropriate public education: The law and children with disabilities* (7th ed.). Denver, CO: Love Publishing Company.

Turnbull, A. P., & Turnbull, H. R. (March–June 2017). *Engaging families and creating trusting partnerships to improve child and family outcomes*. Webinar presented for The Early Childhood Technical Assistance Center.

Turnbull, A. P., Turnbull, H. R., Erwin, E. J., Soodak, L. C., & Shogren, K. A. (2015). *Families, professionals, and exceptionality: Positive outcomes through partnerships and trust*. New York: Pearson.

U. S. Committee for Refugees and Immigrants (n.d.) *Restoring what's been lost*. Retrieved from the USCRI website: http://refugees.org/explore-the-issues/refugees-facts/.

U.S. Bureau of Population, Refugees, and Migration. (February 2018). *U.S. Refugee admissions program FAQs*. Retrieved from: https://www.state.gov/j/prm/releases/factsheets/2018/277838.htm.

U.S. Department of State. (n.d.). *U. S. Refugee admissions program*. Retrieved from: https://www.state.gov/j/prm/ra/admissions/.

UNHCR. (2010). *Convention and protocol related to the status of refugees*. Retrieved from: http://www.unhcr.org/3b66c2aa10.pdf.

UNHCR. (2017). *Global trends: Forced displacement in 2016*. Retrieved from the UNHCR website www.unhcr.org/statistics.

UNHCR. (2018a). *More suffering for the people of Syria*. Retrieved from the UNHCR website: http://www.unhcr.org/sy/.
UNHCR. (2018b). *DR Congo emergency*. Retrieved from the UNHCR website: http://www.unhcr.org/en-us/dr-congo-emergency.html.
Walick, C., & Sullivan, A. L. (2015). Educating Somali immigrant and refugee students: A review of cultural-historical issues and related psychoeducational supports. *Journal of Applied School Psychology, 31*, 1–22.
Walker-Dalhouse, D., & Dalhouse, A. D. (2009). When two elephants fight the grass suffers: Parents and teachers working together to support literacy development of Sudanese youth. *Teaching and Teacher Education, 25*(2), 328–335.
Whitaker, M., & Hoover-Dempsey, K. (2013). School influences on parents' role beliefs. *The Elementary School Journal, 114*(1), 73–99.
Workforce innovation and opportunity Act (WIOA) of 2014. P.L.113-128.
Yohani, S. (2013). Educational cultural brokers and the school adaption of refugee children and families: Challenges and opportunities. *International Migration and Integration, 14*, 61–79. https://doi.org/10.1007/s12134-011-0229-x.

CHAPTER THREE

Supporting Students With Disabilities, Families, and Professionals to Collaborate During the Transition to Adulthood

Grace L. Francis*[,1], Judith M.S. Gross[§], Louise Magiera[§], Joan Schmalzried[§], Amalia Monroe-Gulick[¶] and Sascha Reed*

*George Mason University, Fairfax, VA, United States
[§]Indiana University, Bloomington, IN, United States
[¶]University of Kansas, Lawrence, KS, United States
[1]Corresponding Author: Email: gfranci4@gmu.edu

Contents

International Review of Research in Developmental Disabilities, Volume 54
ISSN 2211-6095
https://doi.org/10.1016/bs.irrdd.2018.07.004

Abstract

Collaboration among students and their families, educators, and service providers is an expectation of secondary transition services for young adults with disabilities. Such collaboration is outlined in special and general education policies, and research demonstrates the positive influence of collaboration on postsecondary outcomes for young adults with disabilities. However, too often, collaboration among these stakeholders does not occur, leaving students and their families struggling to access needed supports after leaving high school. In this chapter, we review the transition planning process, policy related to collaboration and transition planning, and research supporting collaboration during transition to adulthood for young adults with disabilities. We also describe researched transition programs that increase collaboration among students, families, educators and service providers to support successful transitions to adulthood. Implications for practice and future research are discussed.

Transitioning from high school to adulthood is difficult for many young adults with disabilities (U.S. Department of Education, Office of Special Education and Rehabilitative Services, 2017). This is evidenced by low rates of diploma attainment (Hendricks & Wehman, 2009), employment (U.S. Department of Labor, Bureau of Labor Statistics, 2018), participation in postsecondary education or training programs (Grigal, Hart, & Migliore, 2011), and independent living outside of the family home (Hendricks & Wehman, 2009), as compared to young adults without disabilities. For example, the employment rate for working-age individuals with disabilities is 19.7%, versus 65.7% for individuals without disabilities (U.S. Department of Labor, Bureau of Labor Statistics, 2018). However, individualized transition planning and collaboration among students with disabilities, families, and professionals (i.e., educators and adult service providers) can improve positive post-school outcomes of students with disabilities (Haber et al., 2016; Wehman, 2013). The purpose of this manuscript is to review the existing literature on researched transition planning programs and transition activities that increase collaboration among students, families, and professionals to support successful transition outcomes for young adults with disabilities. In the following sections we will: (a) describe the transition planning process for students with disabilities; (b) review theoretical support for student, family, and professional collaboration during transition planning; (c) provide an overview of policies and practices that impact collaboration during transition; (d) describe researched programs and activities designed to increase collaboration among these stakeholders; and (e) present implications for practice and future research.

1. TRANSITION PLANNING PROCESS

Transition planning for students with disabilities is largely driven by federal special education law, the Individuals with Disabilities Education Improvement Act (IDEIA, 2004). According to IDEIA, transition planning is a coordinated set of services for a student that considers the student's strengths and interests and focuses on instruction and experiences that will lead to positive post-school outcomes (2004). Transition planning is required for young adults starting no later than age 16 and must consider planning for postsecondary employment, education/training, and independent living skills. When a student reaches the age of 16 (or earlier), the Individualized Education Program (IEP) becomes guided by transition planning to support the postsecondary goals of the student. The transition-focused IEP is designed to drive student-centered planning and decisions from that point forward. Transition planning under IDEIA is a cyclical process that includes three critical components that support a student's path to postsecondary outcomes. These three components include: (1) age-appropriate transition assessments and a summary of their findings, (2) postsecondary goal statements, and (3) transition services and activities.

1.1 Age-Appropriate Transition Assessments

Along with the student's present levels of academic and functional performance, educators (e.g., teachers, transition specialists, related service providers) conduct annual age-appropriate transition assessments to inform the transition planning process. Though not clearly defined in IDEIA (2004), the Division on Career Development and Transition (DCDT) of the Council for Exceptional Children defines transition assessment as:

> *The ongoing process of collecting data on the individual's needs, preferences, and interests as they relate to the demands of current and future working, educational, living, and personal and social environments. Assessment data serve as the common thread in the transition process [by which IEP teams make decisions] and form the basis for defining goals and services to be included in the Individualized Education Program (IEP)*
>
> ***DCDT (2011)***

Conducting annual age-appropriate transition assessments in the areas of employment, education/training, and independent living support the development of a student's postsecondary goals by identifying interests, skills and preferences, where they currently are on their postsecondary path, and additional skills the student needs to develop in order to achieve their goals.

Age-appropriate transition assessments may be formal or informal (DCDT, 2011). Formal transition assessments provide a structured format for administration and interpretation of transition services, and outcomes of such assessments can be used to compare student data to other students or, in repeated administrations, to the same student over the course of transition planning to demonstrate how participation in transition planning and activities have influenced student goals from year to year. Examples of formal transition assessments include the Transition Planning Inventory, Second Edition (designed to gather information to identify student preferences, needs, and strengths; Patton & Clark, 2014), Student Interest Survey for Career Clusters (designed to isolate student career interests; Advance CTE, n.d.), and the Personal Preference Indicators (designed to identify a student's preferences across numerous domains, including feelings, socialization, and habits; Moss, 2006).

Informal age-appropriate transition assessments are specific to the student and cannot be compared to a standard score or other students' performance (DCDT, 2011). Such assessments are helpful in digging deeper into the student's interests and preferences and gathering information on student participation in various transition activities or services and how that impacts transition planning. Some types of informal assessments include interviews with the student or other significant people (e.g., family members, teachers) and direct observations of the student in community-based activities (e.g., on the job, at home). Another type of informal transition assessment is an "authentic" assessment. Authentic assessments occur when teachers and students take an activity in which the student participated (e.g., welding class, researching colleges, job shadow, community volunteer) and assess its impact on transition planning. For example, if a student chose to take a welding class as an elective, then upon completion of the class, the student and teacher may do an Elective Class Reflection (see appendix for authentic assessment example; Center on Community Living and Careers, 2018c) to assess the impact of the welding class on the student's transition goals. Examples of questions teachers and students may explore during this process may include: Did the student learn more about welding as a potential career? Is the student interested in a career in welding? What skills did the student learn that would help the student to gain employment, be independent, and participate in his/her community? Examples of other authentic assessments in the appendix include a college planning worksheet, a job shadow feedback/reflection, a community service/volunteer experience reflection, and an occupational interview information sheet (Center on Community Living and Careers, 2018a, 2018b, 2018d, 2018e).

1.2 Postsecondary Goal Statements

Once a student has participated in various age-appropriate transition assessments and engaged in meaningful conversations with IEP team members regarding the results, the next part of the transition planning cycle is to support the student in articulating their measurable postsecondary goals, or vision statements. Under IDEIA (2004), measurable postsecondary goals are required in the postsecondary areas of employment and postsecondary education or training, and independent living. Dependent upon a student's age, level of understanding, and experiences, students are often at various stages when determining their postsecondary goal statements. These goals are crafted as "I will" statements and are a way to assist students in thinking about and preparing for their future. Examples of such goals include: "After graduation, I will rent an apartment with a roommate; " "After graduation, I will work 20 or more hours at a garden store with job coaching support; " and "After graduation, I will enroll at the community college and study automotive technology." As with all young adults, postsecondary goal statements often change as students grow, mature, and learn more about themselves and available options. The transition IEP provides the conduit through which families, educators, and service providers can support students as they make informed decisions about their future.

1.3 Transition Services and Activities

After conducting age-appropriate transition assessments and determining measurable postsecondary goal statements, IEP team members identify individualized transition services and activities that are designed to support the student in achieving the postsecondary goals. IDEIA defines transition services as:

> *A coordinated set of activities that are designed to be a results-oriented process, that is focused on improving the academic and functional achievement of the child with a disability to facilitate the child's movement from school to post-school*

> *activities, including post-secondary education, vocational education, integrated employment (including supported employment), continuing and adult education, adult services, independent living, or community participation; and are based on the individual child's needs, taking into account the child's strengths, preferences, and interests …*
>
> ***Sec. 1401(34)***

Examples of transition services and activities include instruction in self-advocacy skills, personal banking, public transportation, personal shopping or hygiene, orientation and mobility, and recreation. Though not all transition services and activities are instruction-based; they may also be experience-based. For example, the student may do a job shadow, volunteer, or work experience with an employer in their field of interest or research the requirements for a college or training program and conduct a college visit with their family. The intention of developing transition services and activities is to provide students with opportunities to gather further information, gain practical experience, or develop a better understanding of the postsecondary goals they have chosen. Therefore, the services and activities identified in the transition plan must be individualized to reflect the student's goals. In short, transition services and activities are designed to support students to make informed decisions about their future. One way to ensure that this occurs is to conduct authentic assessments of the transition services and activities and use that information to support annual planning and goal-setting, thus bringing the transition planning process full circle.

Unfortunately, all transition plans are not created equal (Shogren & Plotner, 2012) and the transition planning process is often marred by numerous barriers, including inadequate communication and lack of family engagement in the transition process (Hetherington, et al., 2010), breakdowns in coordination and collaboration among school and adult service providers (U.S. Government Accountability Office [GAO], 2012), a lack of information or misinformation about available supports and services post-high school (U.S. GAO, 2012; Griffin, McMillan, & Hodapp, 2010; National Association of State Directors of Developmental Disabilities Services & Human Services Research Institute, 2012), and low expectations and poor knowledge across all stakeholders (U.S. GAO, 2012).

Effective transition planning emphasizes early collaboration between educators, service providers, families, and students with disabilities and incorporates evidence-based practices found to improve student outcomes (Test, 2012; Wehman, 2011; Winsor, Butterworth, & Coone, 2011). Despite the expectation that comprehensive IEP teams will collaborate to prepare students with disabilities to live, work, and participate in their communities (U.S. Department of Education, Office of Special Education and Rehabilitative Services, 2017), these key stakeholders often report being unsure how to collaborate and help students achieve positive postsecondary outcomes (Timmons, Hall, Bose, Wolfe, & Winsor, 2011; U.S. GAO, 2012). These barriers contribute to the low realization of inclusive postsecondary outcomes for students with developmental disabilities (Anderson, Larson, & Wuorio, 2011; Grigal et al., 2014; Simonsen & Neubert, 2012).

2. THEORETICAL SUPPORT FOR COLLABORATION DURING TRANSITION

Bronfenbrenner's Person-Process-Context-Time (PPCT) theory of human development explicates how the nature and direction of regular and reciprocal interactions between a person and the individuals, objects, and other aspects of their environment influence a person's development over time (Bronfenbrenner, 2005). The PPCT model highlights the significant impact that a person's characteristics (e.g., motivation, behavior, skills) and key stakeholders who come into direct and ongoing contact with an individual has on their development and outcomes. Key stakeholders during the transition to adulthood include families (e.g., parents, caregivers, siblings), educators (e.g., teachers, transition specialists), and service providers (e.g., vocational rehabilitation counselors, Independent Living Centers, community rehabilitation professionals, case managers). Collaboration among these stakeholders is also essential (Bronfenbrenner, 1979) as educators provide information and transition planning, families serve as a source of aid and guidance, and service providers facilitate access to effective services and resources (Gross & Francis, 2015).

The Taxonomy for Transition Programming 2.0 (Kohler, Gothberg, Fowler, & Coyle, 2016) involves five practice categories:

- Student-focused planning (e.g., developing IEPs, transition planning, students participating in IEP and transition plans)
- Student development (e.g., assessment and data-driven decisions, academic preparation for college and work, life, social, and emotional skills, occupational skills)
- Interagency collaboration (e.g., effective cross-agency communication, collaborative service delivery)

- Family engagement (e.g., participation in transition planning, family needs and support identified)
- Program structure (e.g., transition planning meets individual student needs, transition programs are evaluated based on systematic data systems).

This taxonomy reflects many principles presented in Bronfenbrenner's model of human development during transition to adulthood by reinforcing the importance of student development, student-focused planning, family engagement, and interagency collaboration to ensure positive postsecondary outcomes.

As Bronfenbrenner and the Taxonomy for Transition Programming 2.0 models demonstrate, collaboration among students, families, and professionals is essential to student development and positive outcomes during transition. However, there is limited information on how to execute effective collaboration among these stakeholders during transition planning (Mazzotti, Test, & Mustian, 2012; Morningstar & Mazzotti, 2014; Oertle & Trach, 2007; Test et al., 2009). Pulling from existing collaboration models, Trach (2012) outlined a promising tool, *The Degree of Collaboration for Transition* (DCT), that can be used to assess collaboration during transition. Although not yet thoroughly applied in empirical studies, this tool evaluates transition collaboration activities based on six degrees of collaboration among "representatives," or "designated agency member[s] identified for transition services" (Trach, 2012, p. 42). These degrees of collaboration include:

- Coexistence (e.g., minimal or non-existing interactions among representatives, representatives focus on a single transition activity at a time)
- Networking (e.g., minimal interactions among representatives, representative roles are undefined, representatives make decisions in isolation)
- Cooperation (e.g., representatives share information, representative roles are somewhat defined, representatives make decisions in isolation)
- Coordination (e.g., representatives share information and resources frequently, representative roles are defined, representatives make some decisions together)
- Coalition (e.g., representatives share ideas and resources frequently, all representatives weigh in on decisions)
- Collaboration (e.g., representatives "belong to one system, with frequent communication characterized by mutual trust and consensus is reached on all decisions" p. 42).

The *DCT* tool demonstrates the large variance of collaboration activities, from stakeholders working in isolation to working in partnership where all stakeholders actively provide information and resources and engage in ongoing, shared decision-making. Although not emphasized in Trach's (2012) description of the *DCT*, it is also important to note the bi-directionality of interactions among stakeholders (e.g., stakeholders both providing and receiving communication), as well as how information is delivered and received (e.g., formally, informally; Anderson, Lodish, & Weitz, 1987). Further, as Bronfenbrenner and Kohler et al. note, it is essential that educators, service providers, families, and students with disabilities are all involved in collaboration during transition. Based on these theories and models of collaboration during transition, Fig. 1 represents how stakeholders can collaborate with each other during transition. Where each of these stakeholders overlap with each other (the striped and shaded portions of Fig. 1) represents the collaboration among those stakeholders, or, more

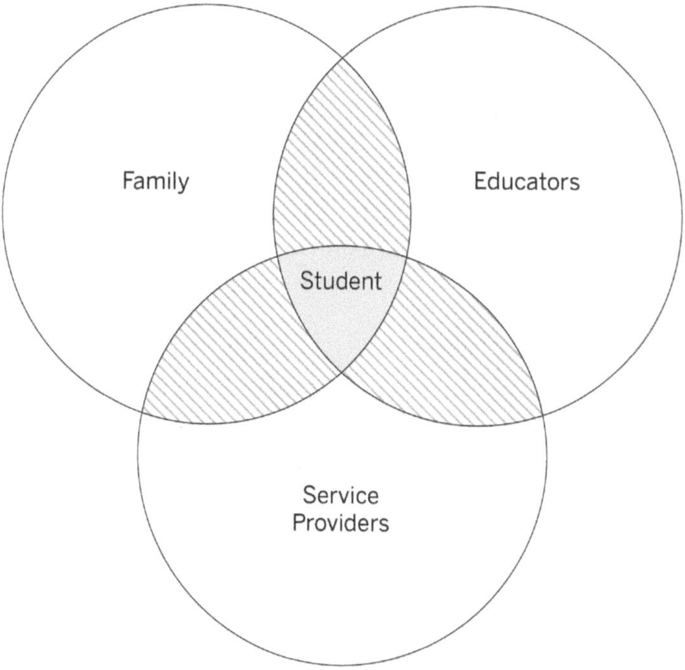

Figure 1 Collaboration among key stakeholders in the transition planning process. This figure illustrates interrelated, bidirectional collaboration across students with disabilities, families, educators, and service providers during transition planning.

specifically, student engagement, family engagement, and interagency collaboration.

Student engagement places students at the center of this system. To be fully engaged during transition, students should, to the greatest degree possible, participate in decision-making and planning with their transition team, work with their families to plan for the future, engage in transition activities and services with educators and service providers, and advocate for their interests and support needs as they work to achieve their postsecondary goals. Family engagement involves families interacting and collaborating with educators and service providers to advocate with and on behalf of their young adults/students. Interagency collaboration involves service providers and educators collaborating with each other to plan and coordinate service provision for the student with disabilities (e.g., transition IEP services, Pre-Employment Transition Services).

3. POLICIES AND PRACTICES THAT IMPACT COLLABORATION AMONG STAKEHOLDERS

Despite discouraging transition outcomes, we know that there are policies and practices related to student engagement, family engagement, and interagency collaboration that are associated with post-school success among individuals with disabilities (Kohler et al., 2016). Discussing policies and practices related to these three constructs will help decipher policy "on the books" and policy "on the streets," (Stowe & Turnbull, 2001, p. 206), as we provide an overview of federal requirements and how they are or are not implemented in practice.

3.1 Student Engagement

Fig. 2 illustrates how student engagement is central to collaboration during transition planning. Transition planning must be student-focused (e.g., student's preferences and goals serve as the basis of transition plans, students are active and contributing members of their planning teams) and support student development (e.g., assessment and development of academic, life, social, occupational and emotional skills, provision of needed services and supports; Kohler et al., 2016). Research demonstrates that when students understand their strengths, interests, preferences, needs, and the IEP process, they have better postsecondary outcomes (Haber, et al., 2016). In order for students to be able to meaningfully participate in the transition planning process, they need support and instruction in

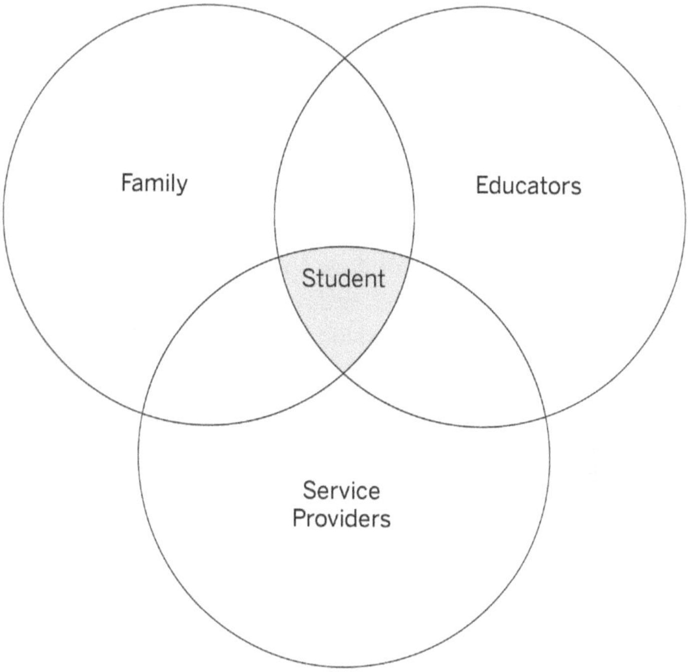

Figure 2 Student engagement during transition planning. This figure illustrates the consistent centrality of student engagement in collaboration among stakeholders during transition planning.

self-determination and decision-making, particularly with respect to understanding the various options that are available to them (Wehmeyer & Shogren, 2013).

Policy. Though the idea of involving students in their transition planning and educational processes has been around for over 50 years, it did not find its way into the Individuals with Disabilities Education Act until 1990 (Martin & Williams-Diehm, 2013). IDEA of 1990 provided the first comprehensive definition of transition planning and instituted the requirement for a transition plan for all students with disabilities starting no later than age 16 (Wehman, 2013). It wasn't until the most recent reauthorization of IDEIA in 2004 that the law required transition IEP monitoring (Indicator 13) and reporting student participation in their educational planning (operationalized as, at a minimum, students being invited to their own IEP meeting by age 16 and participating in age-appropriate transition assessments to support the identification and development of postsecondary goals; IDEIA, 2004; Wehman, 2013).

More recently, the Workforce Innovation and Opportunity Act (WIOA; 2014), which amended the Rehabilitation Act of 1973, expanded vocational rehabilitation services to students through Pre-Employment Transition Services (Pre-ETS). Through the provision of Pre-ETS, students determined eligible or potentially eligible for vocational rehabilitation services have the opportunity to engage in activities that will support them in achieving their postsecondary goals. Required Pre-ETS services under WIOA include job and postsecondary education exploration counseling, work-based learning experiences, and training to develop social skills, independent living skills, and self-advocacy skills [Sec.422(a)(b)(1)(2)(3)(4)]. Examples of Pre-ETS services include students meeting with career counselors to make informed employment-related decisions, job shadowing, engaging in paid or unpaid internships, participating in simulated workplace experiences, engaging in self-advocacy instruction, or peer mentorship.

Practice. Student engagement in the transition process can be accomplished in many ways, including students attending IEPs as well engaging in more active, self-determined practices such as leading their IEP and advocating for their interests and preferences. Several evidence-based practices related to student engagement in the transition process have been developed and researched. Among them, person-centered planning, which focuses on identifying an individual's strengths and planning for the future, has been identified as an effective vehicle for supporting student engagement and collaboration among stakeholders in transition planning (Haines, Francis, Shepherd, Ziegler, & Mabika, 2017; Neece, Kraemer, & Blacher, 2009).

Despite research indicating that practices such as person-centered planning support student engagement in transition planning, students are not often invited to attend or actively participate in their own transition meetings (Agran & Hughes, 2008). In some cases, researchers have found that student-informed transition assessments, services, and goals are nonexistent in transition plans (Martinez, Conroy, & Cerreto, 2012) or, if goals are included in the plan, they do not reflect the goals, needs, and interests of the students for whom they were written (Hetherington et al., 2010). Educators also report being unsure how to help students achieve positive post-secondary outcomes (Timmons et al., 2011; U.S. GAO, 2012). These concerning findings are exacerbated among non-White and non-English speaking students (Antosh et al., 2013; Executive Office of the President, 2014) and students with disabilities who require more significant levels of support (Shogren & Plotner, 2012).

3.2 Family Engagement

Fig. 3 illustrates family engagement with both educators and adult service providers (professionals) during transition planning. Family engagement involves families and professionals regarding each other as reliable allies and providing families with multiple opportunities for meaningful participation (Haines, McCart, & Turnbull, 2013). Families are especially crucial partners to engage in transition planning, as individuals with disabilities who require significant support frequently rely on long-term assistance provided by their families (Developmental Disabilities Act, 2000; Lindstrom, Doren, & Miesch, 2011; Timmons, et al., 2011). Specifically, families influence their members' transition outcomes by modeling positive work ethic, exposing them to a variety of employment (Timmons et al., 2011) and postsecondary education options (Yarbrough, Getzel, & Kester, 2014), establishing expectations for the future and a valorized social role in the community (Boehm, Carter, & Taylor, 2015), and providing guidance and supported-decision making (Neeley-Barnes, Graff,

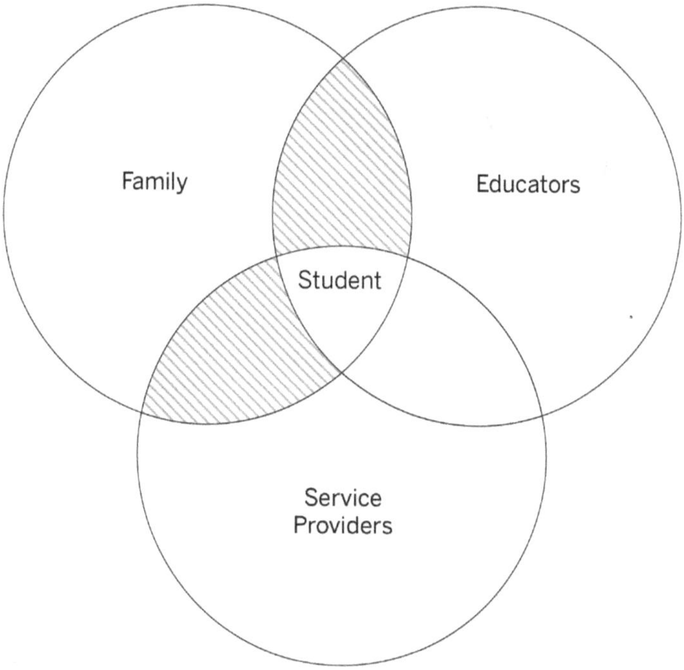

Figure 3 Family engagement in the transition planning process. This figure illustrates how family engagement involves collaboration with professionals during transition planning.

Marcenka, & Weber, 2008). The important role of families in influencing student outcomes (Doren, Gau, & Lindstrom, 2012; Hirano & Rowe, 2015) makes it imperative that they are fully engaged during the transition process and receive support to understand and access services following high school.

Policy. Federal policies address the importance of family engagement through various regulations. For example, the most recent reauthorization of ESSA (2015) included a change in terminology from "parent involvement" to "parent and family engagement," and emphasized the importance of parents making meaningful choices regarding educational services provided to their children [Sec.1003A.(d)(1)(2)]. The statute also mandates that school professionals assist parents to understand topics such as state standards, academic assessments, and how to monitor student progress [Sec.1116(e)(1)] and provide families with materials and training to improve student academic achievement [Sec.1116(e)(2)]. Similarly, IDEIA (2004) includes regulations outlining that "the parents of a child with a disability" [Sec.614.(d)(1)(B)(i)] are essential members of the IEP team who interacts to determine a student's needs, annual goals for the student, and needed services and accommodations that the student requires to receive a free and appropriate education.

IDEIA also allocates federal funding from the U.S. Department of Education to support Parent Training and Information Centers (PTIs) and Community Parent Resource Centers (CPRCs) in every state to better support and inform families of students with disabilities. PTIs and CPRCs provide information and training for families about disability, IDEIA and other relevant laws, and local, state, and national resources to support families and their members with a disability to live, work, and recreate in the community (National Dissemination Center for Children with Disabilities, 2011). PTIs and CPRCs also provide support with advocacy and locating and accessing needed support services. In addition, the Rehabilitation Services Administration (RSA) has provided funding for seven PTIs to provide support to families specifically on issues related to youth transition to adulthood (RAISE Center, 2018).

The Rehabilitation Act of 1973 and its reauthorization the WIOA (2014) reinforce the importance of family engagement through partnering with families as a source of information about and support for the person with a disability, providing funding to support parent information and training, providing services to family members to assist the individual to achieve an employment outcome, and research to support families and individuals with disabilities to better understand and use vocational rehabilitation services and improve the effectiveness of the Rehabilitation Act.

Practice. Engaging families in transition planning can be realized in numerous ways. For example, families can provide information about student strengths and support needs to help professionals to identify resources, which are essential for successful post-school outcomes (Schmidt & Smith, 2007). Other strategies include engaging in ongoing communication, identifying shared resources, acknowledging mutual goals, demonstrating professional competency, and building family leadership (Francis, Blue-Banning, Haines, Turnbull, Gross, 2016; Tonelson & Waters, 1993). Further, in order for family engagement to be successful, transition planning efforts must focus on areas that families value, including information about local services and programs designed to provide direct and ongoing support, family support services, and inclusive community programs (Anderson et al., 2011).

Unfortunately, multiple barriers forestall meaningful family engagement. One predominant barrier includes special educators feeling uncertain how to engage families in the transition process (Lindstrom et al., 2011; Martinez et al., 2012). Given this fact, it is unsurprising that families commonly report being disengaged in IEP meetings (Mueller & Buckley, 2014) and lacking information on transition planning practices, as well as services, supports, and resources available to their students following graduation from high school (Achola & Greene, 2016; Lindstrom et al., 2011; Martinez et al., 2012). In a study conducted by Antosh et al. (2013), over 70% of families of transition-aged students reported needing information on transition planning, and 90% reported needing information on adult services.

Such barriers are exacerbated for families of color and/or who do not speak English as their first language as they report instances of discrimination and poor communication with professionals impacting their ability to participate in transition planning (Francis, Gross, Lavin, Casarez Velazquez, & Sheets, 2018; Hetherington, et al., 2010). Members of culturally diverse families are least responsive to information conveyed through formal meetings or written materials, methods commonly used by transition and employment professionals, leaving them unlikely to participate in transition planning meetings (Geenen et al., 2003) or receive employment services (Hasnain & Balcazar, 2009). Access to and use of employment resources such as formal supports (e.g., vocational rehabilitation, health insurance, job coaching) and informal supports (e.g., family, friends, coworkers, environmental modifications) are positively associated with attainment of competitive employment among culturally and ethnically diverse families (Hasnain & Balcazar, 2009). However, Hispanic, non-Hispanic Black, and Native American youth are less likely than their same age non-Hispanic White peers to have received needed employment services (Executive Office of the President, 2014).

3.3 Interagency Collaboration

Fig. 4 highlights interagency collaboration during transition planning. Interagency collaboration refers to working relationships between educators and service providers (e.g., Vocation Rehabilitation counselors, employment services providers, benefits specialists, independent living counselors, residential support providers, mental health providers) from agencies outside the school system (Kellems & Morningstar, 2010; Kohler et al., 2016).

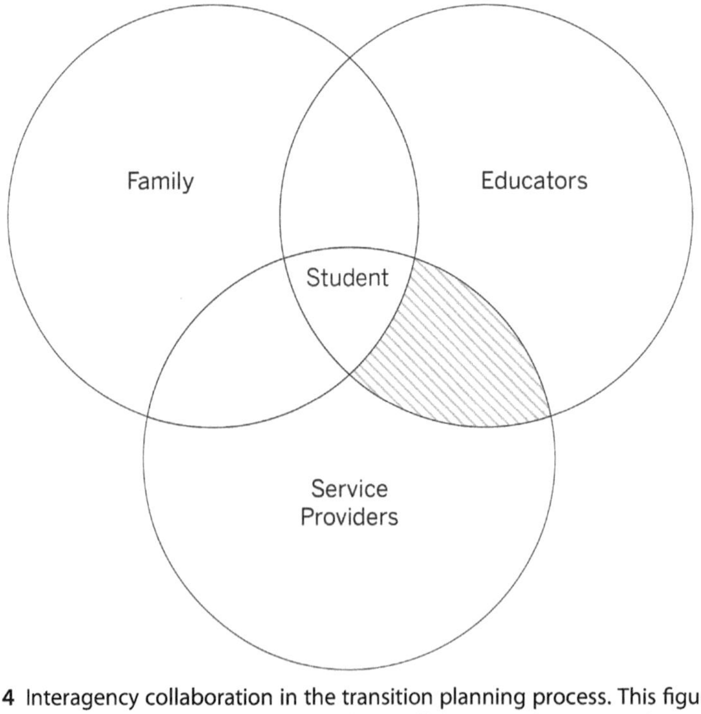

Figure 4 Interagency collaboration in the transition planning process. This figure illustrates how interagency collaboration involves collaboration between educators and service providers during transition planning.

When students with developmental disabilities prepare to finish high school, they typically require or are involved with several different agencies and organizations designed to provide support after graduation. Therefore, interagency collaboration among the service providers from these agencies and organizations is of the utmost importance in order to foster effective and coordinated transition services (AUCD, 2013; Riesen, Schultz, Morgan, & Kupferman, 2014). Two of the primary aims of the transition team are to develop and maintain a fluid transition to adulthood upon leaving the school system and to provide students with several opportunities and choices post-graduation (Kaehne & Beyer, 2009). Effective interagency collaboration can maintain that fluidity and positively influence a student's successful post-school opportunities and outcomes.

Policy. As with student and family engagement, IDEIA (2004) also includes regulations that call for interagency collaboration. According to IDEIA, transition planning should include a "coordinated set of activities" to improve student outcomes following graduation [Sec. 1401(34)]. Further, IDEIA calls for the "development and implementation of transition programs, including coordination of services with agencies involved in supporting the transition of children with disabilities to postsecondary activities" [Sec.611.(e)(2)(C)(vi)]. The statue also notes interagency coordination throughout numerous other sections to ensure "timely and appropriate delivery of services" (including transition services) to students with disabilities [Sec.612(a)(12)(A)(iv)]. Further, WIOA (2014) describes Pre-ETS coordination responsibilities, including service providers attending student IEP or person-centered planning meetings (when invited) and collaborating with other agencies and employers to develop work opportunities for students with disabilities, and service providers and educators carrying out IDEIA transition provisions and WIOA Pre-ETS activities [Sec. 422(d)(1)(2)(3)(4)].

Practice. When students with disabilities prepare to finish high school, they typically require or are involved with several different agencies and organizations designed to provide support after graduation. Therefore, interagency collaboration among the service providers from these agencies and organizations is of the utmost importance in order to foster effective and coordinated transition services (AUCD, 2013; Riesen et al., 2014; U.S. GAO, 2012). Noonan et al. (2008) identified 11 key strategies educators and service providers can use improve interagency collaboration and support students' achievement of successful postsecondary outcomes. These strategies include:

- Providing flexible scheduling and staffing (e.g., providing transition coordinators time and resources to collaborate with stakeholders),
- Following-up after graduation (e.g., collecting follow-up data on student outcomes),
- Providing administrative support for transition (e.g., administrators allowing flexible scheduling, providing professional development, compensating time),
- Using a variety of funding sources (e.g., sharing funding and costs across agencies),
- Utilizing state-supported technical assistance (e.g., state education transition coordinators prioritizing local needs, providing on-going support),
- Building relationships with agencies (e.g., partnering with community service agencies, sharing resources, goal-setting),
- Having meetings with students and their families (e.g., connecting students, families, and service agencies outside of IEP meetings),
- Providing training for students and families (e.g., providing information about service agencies, employment, and post-secondary education),
- Offering joint training opportunities for professionals (e.g., local transition conferences for school and service agency professionals)
- Hosting meeting with school and service agency professionals (e.g., ongoing meetings to share information and problem-solve, goal-setting), and
- Disseminating information to a broad audience (e.g., providing information parents and students about adult service agencies/strategies for securing services, creating manuals, websites, and checklists).

Additional practices include establishing clear roles and responsibilities, sharing data, and coordinating requests for information (Kohler et al., 2016).

Unfortunately, research on interagency collaboration demonstrates a lack of coordination between professionals (Pallisera, Vila, & Fullana, 2014; Plotner, Rose, VanHorn Stinnett, & Ivester, 2017). This shortage of interagency collaboration could arise from several factors, such as a change in staff turnover before the transition plan has been completed, a shortage of adult service provider attendance at collaboration and transition meetings, issues with referral processes, and a lack of knowledge about transition resources (Jen-Yi, Bassett, & Hutchinson, 2009; Kaehne & Beyer, 2009; Plotner et al., 2017; Taylor, Morgan, & Callow-Heusser, 2016). Educators and service providers also report feeling unsure how to collaborate, as well as low levels of satisfaction with the degree to which they collaborate with one another (Jen-Yi et al., 2009; Riesen et al., 2014; Taylor et al., 2016). Insufficient information sharing, a lack of continuity and coordination between school and post-school services, unclear transition procedures, and a lack of leadership are the main problems perceived by professionals that impact successful interagency collaboration (Pallisera, Vilà, & Fullana, 2014).

4. SEARCH AND REVIEW METHODS

In order to gain a better understanding of effective programs that reflect best practice and policy requirements and address barriers commonly found in the research, we searched for researched programs that supported collaboration among key stakeholders (i.e., students, families, educators, and professionals) in student transition to adulthood.

4.1 Search Process

To ensure a broad investigation into programs that support collaboration during transition to adulthood, a social services research librarian searched three library databases (ERIC, PsycInfo, and Pubmed) using language and date filters, along with applicable "subject" or age (focusing on transition age 14–22 years) filters when applicable. The librarian conducted test searches in all three databases to determine the most appropriate terms, including concepts and controlled vocabulary. Searches across databases used disability-specific and transition-specific search terms appropriate for each database. Across the databases, the librarian used up to 31 disability-specific search terms (i.e., names of specific disabilities and general disability terms) along with up to 13 transition-specific search terms (e.g., transition planning, school to work transition, post-school, transition to adulthood, transitional programs). The combined results of this search of three databases resulted in 613 citations across 2003–2017 for review.

4.2 Vetting Process

We used the following inclusionary criteria to vet citations for this chapter: articles that (a) were published in years 2003–2017 in a peer-reviewed journal, (b) targeted at least two of the four collaboration stakeholders discussed in this manuscript (i.e., students with a disability recognized under IDEIA, families, educators, and/or adult service providers; see Fig. 1), and (c) focused on collaboration among the stakeholders. We also employed two exclusionary criteria. First, articles that lacked outcome data on the efficacy of the program on student outcomes were not included for review. Second, since we focused on collaboration as it occurs in a US context (including US policies that guide transition services and supports), articles describing research conducted outside the US were also excluded.

Two university faculty in special education used these criteria to review the search returns. We began by reviewing article titles and abstracts for relevance to transition to adulthood with relation to the population targeted, stakeholders identified as the collaborators, and data collected on the impact of the collaboration. Through this stage of the review, we narrowed the results down to eight articles that met all established criteria.

4.3 Article Review Process

We reviewed the eight remaining articles in full, identifying (a) the name of the collaborative program described, (b) the degree of collaboration employed (Trach, 2012), (c) the key stakeholders involved in the programs, (d) the types of interactions among the key stakeholders involved, and (e) the outcomes for the students participating in the collaborative transition program. See Fig. 5 for a summary of these key elements.

5. TRANSITION PROGRAMS SUPPORTING COLLABORATION

We reviewed eight articles on collaborative transition programs. The first column of Fig. 5 includes an abbreviated reference with the primary author and article title. Column two of Fig. 5 displays the name of the program researched in the article and the general degree of collaboration in which stakeholders engaged described in the research. We used the six degrees of collaboration in Trach's *DCT* tool (2012) to evaluate the transition collaboration activities described in each research article we reviewed. Column three identifies the key stakeholders described in the article. Column four shows the interactions among those stakeholders and the types of collaborative activities that they engaged in together. Finally, column five describes the student outcomes associated with the collaborative transition program described.

In the next section we summarize our findings in the articles reviewed by (a) highlighting commonalities among programs, (b) describing the ways in which collaboration was incorporated as a key element of the programs, and (c) reporting the resulting outcomes for the students involved.

Abbreviated Reference	Program and Degree of Collaboration	Key Stakeholders	Stakeholder Interactions	Student Outcomes
Balcazar, et al. (2012) Improving the Transition Outcomes of Low-income Minority Youth with Disabilities	College Connection Program (CCP) *Coordination:* representatives share information and resources, frequent communication, representative roles are defined, representatives make some decisions together	Students • Young adults with disabilities aged 18-25 years Educators • Special education personnel • College disability support services offices and teachers Adult service providers • Case managers • VR counselors Other • Employers • Business managers or supervisors	• Student-Adult service provider o Goal-setting and developing timelines o Family support and mediation o Emotional support o Referrals to service providers and other services – connecting to services o Transportation training • Adult service provider-Educators o College application support o Curriculum adaptations • Adult service provider-Adult service provider o On-the-job support and monitoring o Job and vocational skill development o Job clubs • Adult service provider-Other o On-the-job support and monitoring	CCP students were significantly more likely than non-attendees to • Secure employment • Earn a higher wage • Participate in a postsecondary education program • Complete a postsecondary education program
Certo, et al. (2003) Review and Discussion of a Model for Seamless Transition to Adulthood	Transition Service Integration Model *Collaboration:* representatives belong to/work as one system, frequent communication, characterized by mutual trust, and consensus is reached on all decisions	Educators • Special education personnel • Administration Adult service providers • Private non-profit agency – vendor for both VR and DD services • VR representative and funding • DD representative and funding	• Educator-Adult service provider o Shared funding o Share office space at the agency o Conduct all planning and scheduling together o Provide all instruction within the community o Participation in policy management group to review progress of participants and resolve policy or service issues	After four years of implementation • 63% of all graduates were employed when exiting school • 88% of all graduates experienced a seamless transition, with no break in support services after leaving school Three-year maintenance research shows that • 90% of graduates were still receiving support from the same non-profit agency • 71% are who were employed at graduation are still employed

Figure 5 Summary of the key elements of collaborative transition programs. This figure outlines the collaborative program and the degree of collaboration according to Trach's (2012) *DCT* tool, identifies key stakeholders in the program, highlights stakeholder interactions, and reports student outcomes. All instances of "VR" indicates "vocational rehabilitation." All instances of "DD" indicates "developmental disabilities" (Abbreviated References: Povenmire-Kirk et al., 2015, Grossi and Thomas, 2017, Cranston-Gingras et al., 2015).

Christensen, et al. (2015)
 	
Longitudinal Outcomes of Project SEARCH in Upstate New York
	Project SEARCH
	
	Coordination: representatives share information and resources, frequent communication, representative roles are defined, representatives make some decisions together
		Students
		• High school students
		• School districts
		• Boards of Cooperative Education Services
		
		Educators
		• Teachers
		• Job coaches
		
		Adult service providers
		• VR staff
		• State DD agency staff
		Other
		• Employers
		• Co_workers
			• Employer-Educator-Adult service provider
			  o Serve on interview and selection committee for program applicants
			
			• Student-Educator-Adult service provider
			  o Support students on the job
			
			• Student-Adult service provider
			  o Job development, search, and support
				For Project SEARCH program completers
				• Average overall rate of employment was 83%
				• Hourly wages ($8.65 to $11.24) and weekly hours worked (23 hours to 35 hours) increased over time
				• From 12-months to 48 months post-graduation, rates of job retention declined to only 44% of program graduates remaining employed at 48 months post.

Cranston-Gingras, et al. (2015)
 	
Going to College: A Campus-Based Partnership for Students with Intellectual Disabilities
	Campus-based transition program
	
	Coalition: representatives share ideas and resources frequently; frequent and prioritized communication; all representatives weigh in on decisions
		Students
		• Young adults with disabilities aged 18-22 years
		
		Family
		
		Educators
		• School district
		• College campus
		
		Other
		• University students
			• Educator-Educator
			  o Transition program became an entity at the college and in the Department of Special Education
			  o College provided a space and operational expenses
			  o School district provided staffing and curriculum
			
			• Family-Student
			  o Provide support for transportation
			  o Provide support using online tools (e.g., email, calendar)
				• 93.6% students received travel training; taking an average of just over four days to successfully master the training
				• 93% participated in at least one internship; over one-third participated in 3 or more
				• 55.5% of the students enrolled in the program were employed within a paid position during their participation in the program
				• 50.8% remained employed in a paid position immediately following their participation

Grossi & Thomas (2017)
 	
Working with Schools: What Employment Providers Need to Know for Successful Collaboration
	Indiana School-to-Work Collaborative
	
	Coalition: representatives share ideas and resources frequently; frequent and prioritized communication; all representatives weigh in on decisions
		Students
		• High school students with disabilities
		
		Educators
		• Transition specialists
		• School representatives
		
		Adult service providers
		• VR staff
		• Community rehabilitation providers
		• Benefits Information Network (BIN) liaisons
		
		Other
		• Employers
		• State Parent Training and Information Center
			• Student-Family-Adult service providers
			  o Helps families to connect with other needed community resources
			  o Provide benefits planning and support to family and student
			
			• Student-Educators
			  o Support the student with communications
			  o Provide self-determination curriculum
			
			• Educators-Adult service providers
			  o Service provider acts as Career Coach and is embedded in the school and focused on access to services and employment
			  o Educators support service providers to understand school culture and practices
			
			• Educators-Adult service providers-Employers
			  o Coordinating internships, work experiences, and paid employment
				After two years of implementation
				• 22% employment rate for students leaving school
				• Average wage of $8.36 (range of $7.25 to $12.40)
				• Average hours worked at 25 per week (range of 5 to 40 hours)
				• Students at collaborative sites were more likely to be connected to adult service providers than students in schools without embedded resources

Figure 5 *(continued)*

Lindstrom et al., (2009)
 	
Building Employment Training Partnerships Between Vocational Rehabilitation and Community Colleges
	Career Workforce Skills Training (CWST)
	
	Coalition: representatives share ideas and resources frequently; frequent and prioritized communication; all representatives weigh in on decisions
		Students
		• Community college students with disabilities
		
		Educators
		• Community college staff
		• University staff
		
		Adult service providers
		• VR services
		• Community rehabilitation providers
		
		Other
		• Employers
			• Educators-Adult service providers
			  o Joint funding
			  o Participation in the local workgroup
			  o Education program research
			
			• Student-Adult service provider
			  o Job development, search, and support
			  o Education program planning
			  o Supported education services to student (e.g., progress monitoring, paperwork completion, timeline management, advocacy, identifying and accessing campus services)
			
			• Educators-Employers
			  o Development of individualized training to meet the interests of the student and needs of employer
				The consumers who participated in the CWST at the college
				• Earned a mean quarterly wage of $9.35 per hour during their first year after leaving the program, compared to $7.89 per hour for non-completers
				• Worked a mean of 291 hours per quarter, compared to 197 for non-completers
				
				The CWST
				• Increased access to college services and activities for students with disabilities on campus
				• Increased collaboration among the community college, VR, and the student

Povenmire-Kirk, et al. (2015)
 	
Implementing CIRCLES: A New Model for Interagency Collaboration in Transition Planning
	Communicating Interagency Relationships and Collaborative Linkages for Exceptional Students (CIRCLES)
	
	Coordination: representatives share information and resources, frequent communication, representative roles are defined, representatives make some decisions together
		Students
		• High school special education students
		
		Family
		
		Educators
		• IEP team comprised of educators and related service providers
		
		Adult service providers
		• Community Level Team (CLT) comprised of disability service provider administrators
		• School Level Team (SLT) comprised of direct service providers from each CLT agency
			• Educators-Adult service providers
			  o CLT team members meet to address policy and practice issues and barriers, identify community needs, and make budgetary considerations
			
			• Adult service providers-Student-Family-Educator
			  o Student presentation of goals
			  o Conduct planning meetings with the SLT to support the student and family to make adult service provider connections and plan for appropriate transition services and supports
			
			• Educators-Student-Family
			  o Teachers incorporate information from SLT meetings into the transition components of the IEP
				Qualitative research with adult service providers who participated in CIRCLES indicated that
				• The SLT facilitated teamwork among agencies to better meet the needs of families and students

Sheppard-Jones, et al. (2007)
 	
Community-based Work Experiences for Students with Significant Disabilities: Real-world Work Equals Real-world Success
	Community-Based Work Transition Program (CBWTP)
	
	Coordination: representatives share information and resources, frequent communication, representative roles are defined, representatives make some decisions together
		Students
		• High school students with disabilities
		
		Family
		
		Educators
		• Special education staff
		
		Adult service providers
		• VR services
		• Community rehabilitation providers
		
		Other
		• Employers
			• Educators-Adult service providers
			  o School districts and VR pooled resources and provided VR services before students graduated
			
			• Student-Family-Educator-Adult service provider
			  o Developed IEP and IPE for student to guide transition service delivery
				Two years after exiting high school
				• 69% of participants who had a closed VR case following participation in the CBWTP were successfully employed, as compared to only 45.6% of the general VR population at the time

Figure 5 ***(continued)***

5.1 Commonalities Among Programs

The most commonly identified collaborative stakeholders in the articles we reviewed were educators and service providers. The collaborative activities in which these stakeholders engaged ranged from simple referrals for services, to joint planning, funding, resource sharing, and service delivery (see Fig. 5). The most commonly identified service providers were vocational rehabilitation counselors or other vocational rehabilitation staff, followed by community rehabilitation professionals and developmental disabilities service providers.

The least commonly identified stakeholders were families. When families were identified as a stakeholder, their role was generally described in terms of providing student support (e.g., transportation, assistance with use of electronic communications) or assisting to identify postsecondary goals and transition services and activities. Further, although some programs noted more self-determined forms of student engagement through activities such as connecting with service providers and applying and practicing skills (e.g., Balcazar et al., 2012; Lindstrom, Flannery, Benz, Olszewski, & Slovic, 2009), student engagement activities commonly reflected lower degrees of collaboration, including students responding to questions, providing input on interests, and receiving services and instruction.

Other commonalities among these programs included that the schools and adult service agencies in five of the programs pooled funding or other resources (e.g., office or classroom space, staffing), three of the programs were housed on community college and university campuses (with an emphasis on students attaining both education and employment outcomes), and all but two programs specifically identified state vocational rehabilitation services and staff as key partners (see Fig. 5). In the following section we highlight robust descriptions and exemplars of unique collaborative transition activities.

5.2 Degrees of Collaboration and Student Outcomes Among Programs

In order to better identify the different degrees of collaboration described in the research reviewed, we assigned each article one of Trach's (2012) six degrees of collaboration by focusing on the highest level of collaborative activities described in the article. According to Trach's ranking of degrees of collaboration, the eight articles we reviewed represented the three highest degrees of collaboration (see Fig. 5): *coordination* ($n = 4$), *coalition* ($n = 3$), and true *collaboration* ($n = 1$).

Coordination. *Coordination* (identified in four articles) was the most commonly represented degree of collaboration and was characterized by clearly defined roles among stakeholders, information and resource sharing, frequent communication, and occasional shared decision-making. We highlight one example, the College Connection Program described by Balcazar et al. (2012) which involved a case manager working with transition stakeholders (i.e., students with a disability, educators at the high school and community college, service providers, and employers and supervisors) to make connections among the stakeholders and coordinate all services and supports in alignment with the student's postsecondary goals. This program also focused on student-centered services and supports across school and work environments, coordinated by the case manager. This level of intensive support resulted in improved outcomes for students, with program attendees being more likely to secure employment, earn a higher wage, and complete a postsecondary education or training program.

Other programs using a *coordination* degree of collaboration such as Project SEARCH participants (Christensen, Hetherington, Daston, & Riehle, 2015) and Community-Based Work Transition Program participants (Sheppard-Jones, Garrett, & Huff, 2007) experienced similar results. Findings from these programs indicated that students attained employment at higher rates and earned increasingly higher wages and working more hours over time than individuals receiving traditional transition services without the emphasis on *coordination*.

Coalition. *Coalition* (identified in three articles) was the next most common degree of collaboration and was characterized by the sharing of ideas and resources with frequent and prioritized communication among stakeholders and all stakeholders weighing in on decisions. We highlight one program described by Lindstrom et al. (2009) which provided a clear example of *coalition* in their description of the Career Workforce Skills Training (CWST) program. In this program, vocational rehabilitation staff and a college combined funds to pay for an employment specialist to work with students who were referred to the college by vocational rehabilitation to receive short-term skills training for a specific employment opportunity. This employment specialist worked with students in job development as well as provided supported education services (e.g., progress monitoring, paperwork completion, timeline management, advocacy, identifying and accessing campus services) to ensure that students had the support they needed to successfully complete the training program. Educators worked with potential employers, students, and the employment specialist to develop individualized trainings to meet the needs of students and employers. Students who completed the program earned more per hour and worked more hours per quarter than those who did not complete the program. In addition, the program also increased access to college services and activities for students.

True collaboration. True *collaboration* (identified in one article) was characterized by stakeholders working as a single unit, frequent communication characterized by mutual trust, and consensus being reached among stakeholders. The Transition Service Integration Model described by Certo et al. (2003) reflected this degree of collaboration by focusing on integrating the services of special education, developmental disabilities, and vocational rehabilitation prior to students leaving secondary school in order to ensure that students had a seamless transition with no break in services or supports. In this program, the key stakeholders included educators and service providers. The program was a community immersion program, where all instruction took place in the community. Through shared funding and resources, the educator and service provider (who was a vendor for both vocational rehabilitation and developmental disabilities services through the state) shared an office space in the service provider's agency located in the community. These stakeholders conducted all planning and scheduling together and provided all instruction in the community. At three years following program participation, 71% of the students who had gained employment were still employed, and nearly all were still receiving support from the same agency.

6. IMPLICATIONS FOR PRACTICE

The programs we reviewed primarily reflected the three highest degrees of collaboration according to Trach's (2012) *DCT* tool: *coordination* ($n = 4$), *coalition* ($n = 3$), and *collaboration* ($n = 1$). Although collaboration during transition planning is not always easy due to several barriers (e.g., funding limitations, a lack of knowledge of who should be part of the transition planning team, distrust, and communication barriers; Achola & Greene, 2016; Lindstrom et al., 2011; Timmons et al., 2011), our analysis suggests that stakeholders can use collaborative strategies such as sharing personnel, physical resources and spaces, and funding to support student outcomes during transition (see Fig. 5). These articles also highlighted the importance of shared decision-making and planning to achieve true collaboration among all stakeholders during transition.

We analyzed the transition programs featured in each article as a whole by assigning a degree of collaboration based on the highest degree described in each program. However, as noted in the "Commonalities Among Programs" section, there were many interactions among stakeholders that did not reflect these higher-order degrees of collaboration. For example, family engagement and student activities generally reflected a lower level of collaboration - *cooperation*-with their roles limited to sharing and receiving information and a having a defined role (e.g., providing students support, students receiving support), instead of engaging in shared-decision making (see Fig. 5). Moreover, the most commonly identified service providers were vocational rehabilitation counselors or other vocational rehabilitation staff, followed by community rehabilitation professionals and developmental disabilities service providers. This narrow focus on specific professionals is not representative of the numerous community representatives that may play meaningful roles during transition planning.

It is essential that transition teams think beyond common transition practices and players, and carefully consider how to maximize student and family engagement and interagency collaboration. For example, depending on a student's needs, transition stakeholders should expand to include individuals such as school or service agency administrators, social workers, independent living counselors, cultural liaisons, and mental health providers. In addition, several articles reviewed in chapter noted employers as a transition stakeholder (see Fig. 5). Some ways in which employers were included as transition stakeholders included participating on interview committees and collaborating with educators to develop a job training curriculum (Christensen et al., 2015; Lindstrom et al., 2009). Increasing such opportunities to enhance the variety of stakeholders involved in transition programs, including employers, and the ways in which they collaborate will likely to contribute to successful postsecondary outcomes of students with disabilities.

Trach's model (2012) for distinguishing degrees of collaboration is helpful for defining expectations for stakeholders in transition planning. However, Trach's *DCT* tool narrowly focuses on interagency collaboration (e.g., collaboration between school and service agency professionals).

This narrow focus was reinforced in the transition program descriptions in many of the articles reviewed (see Fig. 5). However, it is essential that transition teams focus on fully engaging students with disabilities and their families in order to maximize input from all stakeholders to ensure positive student outcomes. This may mean employing additional strategies such as meeting students and families in their homes or communities (Francis, Haines, & Nagro, 2017); learning about student and family cultures, experiences, and expectations (Francis et al., 2017); identifying and addressing student and family barriers (Francis, Gross, Lavin, Casarez, & Sheets, 2018), and using resources such as those identified by Sánchez Gosnell, Mattson, Hernandez, and Saroughi (2018) to engage and support disenfranchised populations, including immigrants (e.g., United We Dream, Welcome to USA.gov). These strategies could mitigate professionals feeling unprepared to collaborate with culturally and linguistically diverse families (Kalyanpur & Harry, 2012) and potentially diminish the stigma and discrimination that individuals with disabilities often experience from employers (Morgan & Alexander, 2005) and other members of their communities (National Disability Rights Network, 2011). In some cases, transition stakeholders may need to invest time and effort to rebuild trusting relationships before collaboration can occur. This many include implementing conflict prevention and resolution practices (Mueller, Singer, & Draper, 2008).

7. DIRECTIONS FOR FUTURE RESEARCH

Future research on interagency collaboration in transition should focus efforts on developing and testing interventions that facilitate all stakeholders' engagement in meaningful, frequent, bidirectional communication. Further, collaborative transition programs should emphasize and provide strategies for stakeholders to engage in shared decision-making, as well as sharing responsibilities to support positive transition outcomes. The stakeholders featured in the studies we reviewed primarily included educators and service providers. It is imperative that future research investigate the collaborative role of additional stakeholders such as community organizations (e.g., parks and recreations, social services, refugee resettlement organizations), community employers, and historically marginalized students and families, as well as how best to develop meaningful, culturally responsive, collaborative relationships with members of diverse transition planning teams.

In that same vein, future research should also focus on how to more meaningfully engage students with significant support needs in their own transition planning. In the articles we reviewed, students' collaborative role was generally limited to that of a receiver of supports and services, as opposed to an active contributor and collaborator in the transition process. While there is much research on self-determination and student led IEPs, there needs to be an increased focus on the role of the young adult as a collaborator and contributor in the implementation of the transition plan.

Finally, future research should consider the long-term impacts and sustainability of collaboration strategies and how to scale-up those practices that have been found effective. While few researchers have used the *DCT* measure in empirical studies, future research could use this tool to determine a baseline of collaboration among stakeholders during transition and as a measure of the impact of interventions such as those described above. Collaboration among all partners in transition can make an impactful difference on the outcomes for youth with developmental disabilities, and such research would support and encourage efforts to ensure that practice aligns with policy.

REFERENCES

Achola, E. O., & Greene, G. (2016). Person-family centered transition planning: Improving post-school outcomes to culturally diverse youth and families. *Journal of Vocational Rehabilitation, 45*, 173–183. https://doi.org/10.3233/JVR-160821.

Advance C.T.E., n.d. Student Interest Survey for Career Cluster. Retrieved from: https://careertech.org/student-interest-survey.

Agran, M., & Hughes, C. (2008). Asking student input: Students' opinions regarding their individualized education program involvement. *Career Development for Exceptional Children, 31*, 69–76. https://doi.org/10.1177/0885728808317657.

Anderson, L., Larson, S. A., & Wuorio, A. (2011). *2010 FINDS national Survey: Family and individual needs for disability Supports: Technical report Part 1*. Minneapolis, MN: Research and Training Center on Community Living, University of Minnesota.

Anderson, E., Lodish, L. M., & Weitz, B. A. (1987). Resource allocation behavior in conventional channels. *Journal of Marketing Research, 24*, 85–97. https://doi.org/10.2307/3151756.

Antosh, A. A., Blair, M., Edwards, K., Goode, T., Hewitt, A., Izzo, M., … Wehmeyer, M. (April 2013). *A collaborative interagency, interdisciplinary approach to transition from adolescence to adulthood*. Silver Spring, MD: Association of University Centers on Disabilities.

AUCD. (2013). *A collaborative interagency, interdisciplinary approach to transition from adolescence to adulthood*. Retrieved from: https://www.aucd.org/docs/publications/transition2013_full_sm2.pdf.

Balcazar, F. E., Taylor-Ritzler, T., Dimpfl, S., Portillo-Peña, N., Guzman, A., Schiff, R., & Murvay, M. (2012). Improving the transition outcomes of low-income minority youth with disabilities. *Exceptionality, 20*, 114–132. https://doi.org/10.1080/09362835.2012.670599.

Boehm, T. L., Carter, E. W., & Taylor, J. L. (2015). Family quality of life during the transition to adulthood for individuals with intellectual disability and/or autism spectrum disorders. *American Journal on Intellectual and Developmental Disabilities, 120,* 395–411. https://doi.org/10.1352/1944-7558-120.5.395.

Bronfenbrenner, U. (1979). *The ecology of human development: Experiments by nature and design.* Thousand Oaks, CA: Sage.

Bronfenbrenner, U. (2005). *Making human being human: Bioecological perspectives on human Development.* Cambridge, MA: Harvard University Press.

Center on Community Living and Careers (CCLC). (2018a). *College planning worksheet.* Retrieved from: https://instrc.indiana.edu/pdf/transition_matrix/AA%20College%20Planning%20Worksheet.pdf.

Center on Community Living and Careers (CCLC). (2018b). *Community service/volunteer experience reflection.* Retrieved from: https://instrc.indiana.edu/pdf/transition_matrix/AA%20Volunteer%20Experience%20Sheet.pdf.

Center on Community Living and Careers (CCLC). (2018c). *Elective class reflection.* Retrieved from: https://instrc.indiana.edu/pdf/transition_matrix/AA%20Elective%20Class%20Reflection.pdf.

Center on Community Living and Careers (CCLC). (2018d). *Job shadow feedback/reflection.* Retrieved from: https://instrc.indiana.edu/pdf/transition_matrix/AA%20Job%20Shadow%20Feedback.pdf.

Center on Community Living and Careers (CCLC). (2018e). *Occupational interview information sheet.* Retrieved from: https://instrc.indiana.edu/pdf/transition_matrix/AA%20Occupational%20Interview%20Information.pdf.

Certo, N. J., Mautz, D., Pumpian, I., Sax, C., Smalley, K., Wade, H. A., … Batterman, N. (2003). Review and discussion of a model for seamless transition to adulthood. *Education and Training in Developmental Disabilities, 38*(1), 3–17. Retrieved from: http://www.jstor.org/stable/23880183.

Christensen, J. J., Hetherington, S., Daston, M., & Riehle, E. (2015). Longitudinal outcomes of Project SEARCH in upstate New York. *Journal of Vocational Rehabilitation, 42,* 247–255. https://doi.org/10.3233/JVR-150746.

Cranston-Gingras, A., Davis, D., Gonzalez, G., Knollman, G., Thomas, D., & Wissner, A. (2015). Going to college: A campus-based partnership for students with intellectual disabilities. *School-university Partnerships, 8*(2), 62–71.

Developmental disabilities assistance and bill of Rights Act (DD Act), 42 U.S.C. § 15001.(2000).

Division on Career Development in Transition (DCDT). (2011). *Age-appropriate transition assessment.* Retrieved from: http://community.cec.sped.org/dcdt/publications/fast-facts.

Doren, B., Gau, J. M., & Lindstrom, L. E. (2012). The relationship between parent expectations and postschool outcomes of adolescents with disabilities. *Exceptional Children, 79,* 7–23. https://doi.org/10.1177/001440291207900101.

Every student succeeds Act (ESSA), 20 U.S.C.§ 1177.(2015).

Executive Office of the President. (December 2014). *2014 Native youth report.* Washington, DC: The White House. Retrieved from: https://obamawhitehouse.archives.gov/sites/default/files/docs/20141129nativeyouthreport_final.pdf.

Francis, G. L., Blue-Banning, M., Haines, S. J., Turnbull, A. P., & Gross, J. M. S. (2016). Building "our school:" Parental perspectives for building trusting family-professional partnerships. *Preventing School Failure, 60,* 329–336. https://doi.org/10.1080/1045988X.2016.1164115.

Francis, G. L., Gross, J. M. S., Lavín, C., Casarez, L., & Sheets, N. (2018). Hispanic caregiver experiences supporting positive post-school outcomes for young adults with disabilities. *Intellectual and Developmental Disabilities* (in press).

Francis, G. L., Haines, S. J., & Nagro, S. A. (2017). Developing relationships with immigrant families: Learning by asking the right questions. *TEACHING Exceptional Children, 50*, 95–105. https://doi.org/10.1177/0040059917720778.

Geenen, S. J., Powers, L., Lopez-Vasquez, A., & Bersani, H. (2003). Understanding and promoting the transition of minority adolescents. *Career Development for Exceptional Individuals, 26*, 27–46. https://doi.org/10.1177/088572880302600103.

Griffin, M. M., McMillan, E. D., & Hodapp, R. M. (2010). Family perspectives on post-secondary education for students with intellectual disabilities. *Education and Training in Autism and Developmental Disabilities, 45*(3), 339–346.

Grigal, M., Hart, D., & Migliore, A. (2011). Comparing the transition planning, postsecondary education, and employment outcomes of students with intellectual and other disabilities. *Career Development for Exceptional Individuals, 34*, 4–17. https://doi.org/10.1177/0885728811399091.

Grigal, M., Hart, D., Smith, F. A., Domin, D., Sulewski, J., & Weir, C. (2014). *Think College National Coordinating Center: Annual report on the transition and postsecondary programs for students with intellectual disabilities (2012–2013)*. Boston, MA: University of Massachusetts Boston, Institute for Community Inclusion.

Gross, J. M. S., & Francis, G. L. (2015). Role of expectations and knowledge in transition to employment. In *Way leads on to Way: Paths to employment for people with intellectual disability* (pp. 63–84). Washington, DC: American Association on Intellectual and Developmental Disabilities.

Grossi, T., & Thomas, F. (2017). Working with schools: What employment providers need to know for successful collaboration. *Journal of Vocational Rehabilitation, 46*, 355–359. https://doi.org/10.3233/JVR-170872.

Haber, M. G., Mazzotti, V. L., Mustian, A. L., Rowe, D. A., Bartholomew, A. L., Test, D. W., & Fowler, C. H. (2016). What works, when, for whom, and with whom: A meta-analytic review of predictors of postsecondary success for students with disabilities. *Review of Educational Research, 86*, 123–162. https://doi.org/10.3102/0034654315583135.

Haines, S. J., Francis, G. L., Shepherd, K., Ziegler, M., & Mabika, G. (2017). Partnership bound: Using MAPS with transitioning students and families from all backgrounds. *Career Development and Transition for Exceptional Individuals*, 1–5. https://doi.org/10.1177/2165143417698123.

Haines, S. J., McCart, A., & Turnbull, A. P. (2013). Family engagement within early childhood Response to Intervention. In V. Buysse, & E. Peisner-Feinberg (Eds.), *Handbook on response to intervention (RTI) in early childhood* (pp. 313–324). New York: Paul H. Brookes.

Hasnain, R., & Balcazar, F. (2009). Predicting community- versus facility-based employment for transition-aged young adults with disabilities: The role of race, ethnicity, and support systems. *Journal of Vocational Rehabilitation, 31*, 175–188. https://doi.org/10.3233/JVR-2009-0487.

Hendricks, D. R., & Wehman, P. (2009). Transition from school to adulthood for youth with autism spectrum disorders: Review and recommendations. *Focus on Autism and Other Developmental Disabilities, 24*, 77–88. https://doi.org/10.1177/1088357608329827.

Hetherington, S. A., Durant-Jones, L., Johnson, K., Nolan, K., Smith, E., Taylor-Brown, S., & Tuttle, J. (2010). The lived experiences of adolescents with disabilities and their parents in transition planning. *Focus on Autism and Other Developmental Disabilities, 25*, 163–172. https://doi.org/10.1177/1088357610373760.

Hirano, K. A., & Rowe, D. A. (2015). A conceptual model for parent involvement in secondary special education. *Journal of Disability Policy Studies, 27*, 43–53. https://doi.org/10.1177/1044207315583901.

Individuals with disabilities education improvement Act (IDEIA). 20 U.S.C. § 1400.(2004).
Jen-Yi, L., Bassett, D. S., & Hutchinson, S. R. (2009). Secondary special educators' transition involvement. *Journal of Intellectual & Developmental Disability, 34*, 163–172. https://doi.org/10.1080/13668250902849113.
Kaehne, A., & Beyer, S. (2009). Views of professionals on aims and outcomes of transition for young people with learning disabilities. *British Journal of Learning Disabilities, 37*(2), 138–144. https://doi.org/10.1111/j.1468-3156.2008.00534.x.
Kalyanpur, M., & Harry, B. (2012). *Cultural reciprocity in special education: Building family-professional relationships*. Baltimore, MD: Brookes.
Kellems, R. O., & Morningstar, M. E. (2010). Tips for transition. *Teaching Exceptional Children, 43*, 60–68. https://doi.org/10.1177/004005991204400502.
Kohler, P. D., Gothberg, J. E., Fowler, C., & Coyle, J. (2016). *Taxonomy for transition programming 2.0: A model for planning, organizing, and evaluating transition education, services, and programs*. Western Michigan University. Available at: www.transitionta.org.
Lindstrom, L., Doren, B., & Miesch, J. (2011). Waging a living: Career development and long-term employment outcomes for young adults with disabilities. *Exceptional Children, 77*, 423–434. https://doi.org/10.1177/001440291107700403.
Lindstrom, L. E., Flannery, K. B., Benz, M. R., Olszewski, B., & Slovic, R. (2009). Building employment training partnerships between Vocational Rehabilitation and community colleges. *Rehabilitation Counseling Bulletin, 52*, 189–201. https://doi.org/10.1177/0034355208323946.
Martinez, D. C., Conroy, J. W., & Cerreto, M. C. (2012). Parent involvement in the transition process of children with intellectual disabilities: The influence of inclusion on parent desires and expectations for postsecondary education. *Journal of Policy and Practice in Intellectual Disabilities, 9*, 279–288. https://doi.org/10.1111/jppi.12000.
Martin, J. E., & Williams-Diehm, K. (2013). Student engagement and leadership of the transition planning process. *Career Development and Transition for Exceptional Individuals, 36*, 43–50. https://doi.org/10.1177/2165143413476545.
Mazzotti, V. L., Test, D. W., & Mustian, A. L. (2012). Secondary transition evidence-based practices and predictors: Implications for policymakers. *Journal of Disability Policy Studies, 35*, 5–18. https://doi.org/10.1177/1044207312460888.
Morgan, R. L., & Alexander, M. (2005). The employer's perception: Employment of individuals with developmental disabilities. *Journal of Vocational Rehabilitation, 23*, 39–49. Retrieved from: https://content.iospress.com/articles/journal-of-vocational-rehabilitation/jvr00295.
Morningstar, M., & Mazzotti, V. (2014). *Teacher preparation to deliver evidence-based transition planning and services to youth with disabilities*. Retrieved from: http://ceedar.education.ufl.edu/tools/innovation-configurations/.
Moss, J. (2006). *Personal preference Indicators: A guide for planning*. Retrieved from: https://www.ou.edu/content/dam/Education/documents/personal-preference-indicator.pdf.
Mueller, T. G., & Buckley, P. C. (2014). The odd man out: How fathers navigate the special education system. *Remedial and Special Education, 35*, 40–49. https://doi.org/10.1177/0741932513513176.
Mueller, T. G., Singer, G. H. S., & Draper, L. M. (2008). Reducing parental dissatisfaction with special education in two school districts: Implementing conflict prevention and alternative dispute resolution. *Journal of Educational and Psychological Consultation, 18*, 191–233. https://doi.org/10.1080/10474410701864339.
National Association of State Directors of Developmental Disabilities Services, & Human Services Research Institute. (2012). *National core Indicators annual summary report 2010–2011*. Retrieved from: https://www.hsri.org/publication/nci-annual-summary-report-2010-2011.

National Disability Rights Network. (2011). *Segregated and exploited: A call to action.* Retrieved from: http://www.ndrn.org/images/Documents/Resources/Publications/Reports/Segregated-and-Exploited.pdf.
National Dissemination Center for Children with Disabilities. (January 2011). *PTIs and CPRCs: Resources for parents.* Retrieved from: https://www.parentcenterhub.org/wp-content/uploads/repo_items/bp3.pdf.
Neece, C. L., Kraemer, B. R., & Blacher, J. (2009). Transition satisfaction and family well being among parents of young adults with severe intellectual disability. *Intellectual and Developmental Disabilities, 47*, 31–43. https://doi.org/10.1352/2009.47:31-43.
Neeley-Barnes, S., Graff, J. C., Marcenka, M., & Weber, L. (2008). Family decision making: Benefits to persons with developmental disabilities and their family members. *Intellectual and Developmental Disabilities, 46*, 93–105. https://doi.org/10.1352/0047-6765.
Noonan, P. M., Morningstar, M. E., & Erickson-Gaumer, A. (2008). Improving interagency collaboration: Effective strategies used by high-performing local districts and communities. *Career Development for Exceptional Individuals, 31*, 132–143. https://doi.org/10.1177/0885728808327149.
Oertle, K. M., & Trach, J. S. (2007). Interagency collaboration: The importance of rehabilitation professionals' involvement in transition. *Journal of Rehabilitation, 73*(3), 36–44.
Pallisera, M., Vilà, M., & Fullana, J. (2014). Transition to adulthood for young people with intellectual disability: Exploring transition partnerships from the point of view of professionals in school and postschool services. *Journal of Intellectual & Developmental Disability, 39*, 333–341. https://doi.org/10.3109/13668250.2014.938032.
Patton, J. R., & Clark, G. M. (2014). *TPI-2: Transition planning inventory* (2nd ed.) Retrieved from: https://www.mhs.com/MHS-Assessment?prodname=TPI-2.
Plotner, A., Rose, C., VanHorn Stinnett, C., & Ivester, J. (2017). Professional characteristics that impact perceptions of successful transition collaboration. *Journal of Rehabilitation, 83*(2), 43–51.
Povenmire-Kirk, T., Dieglemann, K., Crump, K., Schnorr, C., Test, D., Flowers, C., & Aspel, N. (2015). Implementing CIRCLES: A new model for interagency collaboration in transition planning. *Journal of Vocational Rehabilitation, 42*, 51–65. https://doi.org/10.1177/0022466917720764.
RAISE Center. (2018). *RSA parent centers.* Retrieved from: http://www.raisecenter.org/rsa-parent-centers/.
Rehabilitation Act, 29 U.S.C., § *701.*(1973).
Riesen, T., Schultz, J., Morgan, R., & Kupferman, S. (2014). School-to-work barriers as identified by special educators, vocational rehabilitation counselors, and community rehabilitation professionals. *Journal of Rehabilitation, 80*(1), 33–44.
Sánchez Gosnell, E. S., Mattson, J., Hernandez, D., & Saroughi, M. (2018). Resources for allies, activists, and advocates for immigrant children and their families. In S. Wong, E. Sánchez Gosnell, A. M. Foerster Luu, & L. Dodson (Eds.), *Teachers as Allies: Transformative practices for teaching DREAMers and undocumented students* (pp. 170–183). New York, NY: Teachers College Press.
Schmidt, M. A., & Smith, D. L. (2007). Individuals with disabilities perceptions on preparedness for the workforce and factors that limit employment. *Work: a Journal of Prevention, Assessment, and Rehabilitation, 28*(1), 13–21.
Sheppard-Jones, K., Garrett, B., & Huff, M. B. (2007). Community-based work experiences for students with significant disabilities: Real-world work equals real-world success. *International Journal on Disability and Human Development, 6*, 47–52. https://doi.org/10.1515/IJDHD.2007.6.1.47.
Shogren, K. A., & Plotner, A. J. (2012). Characteristics of transition planning for students with intellectual disability, autism or other disabilities: Data from the National Longitudinal Transition Study-2. *Intellectual and Developmental Disabilities, 50*, 16–30. https://doi.org/10.1352/1934-9556-50.1.16.

Simonsen, M. L., & Neubert, D. A. (2012). Transitioning youth with intellectual and other developmental disabilities: Predicting community employment outcomes. *Career Development and Transition for Exceptional Individuals, 36*, 188–198. https://doi.org/10.1177/2165143412469399.

Stowe, M. J., & Turnbull, H. R. (2001). Tools for analyzing policy "on the books" and policy "on the streets". *Journal of Disability Policy Studies, 12*(3), 106–214.

Taylor, D. L., Morgan, R. L., & Callow-Heusser, C. A. (2016). A survey of vocational rehabilitation counselors and special education teachers on collaboration in transition planning. *Journal of Vocational Rehabilitation, 44*, 163–173. https://doi.org/10.3233/JVR-150788.

Test, D. W. (2012). *Evidence-based instructional strategies for transition*. Baltimore, MD: Paul Brookes Publishing.

Test, D. W., Mazzotti, V. L., Mustian, A. L., Fowler, C. H., Kortering, L., & Kohler, P. (2009). Evidence-based secondary transition predictors for improving postschool outcomes for students with disabilities. *Career Development for Exceptional Individuals, 32*, 160–181. https://doi.org/10.1177/0885728809346960.

Timmons, J. C., Hall, A. C., Bose, J., Wolfe, A., & Winsor, J. (2011). Choosing employment: Factors that impact employment decisions for individuals with intellectual disability. *Intellectual and Developmental Disabilities, 49*(4), 285–299.

Tonelson, S. W., & Waters, R. (1993). Interagency collaboration. In B. Billingsly (Ed.), *Program leadership in special education* (pp. 55–66). Richmond, VA: Virginia Department of Education.

Trach, J. S. (2012). Degree of collaboration for successful transition outcomes. *Journal of Rehabilitation, 78*(2), 39–48.

U.S. Department of Education, Office of Special Education and Rehabilitative Services (USED, OSERS). (2017). *A transition guide to postsecondary education and employment for students and youth with disabilities*. Washington, D.C.: Author.

U.S. Department of Labor, Bureau of Labor Statistics. (2018). *Table A-6. Employment status of the civilian population by sex, age, and disability status, not seasonally adjusted*. Retrieved from: http://www.bls.gov/news.release/empsit.t06.htm.

U.S. Government Accountability Office (GAO). (2012). *Students with disabilities: Better federal coordination could lessen challenges in the transition from high school*. Report to the Ranking Member, Committee on Education and the Workforce, House of Representatives (GAO-12–594). Available at: http://www.eric.ed.gov/ERICWebPortal/detail?accno=ED534179.

Wehman, P. (2011). *Essentials of transition planning*. Baltimore, MD: Paul Brookes Publishing.

Wehman, P. (2013). Transition: New horizons and challenges. In P. Wehman (Ed.), *Life beyond the classroom: Transition strategies for young people with disabilities* (5th ed., pp. 3–40). Baltimore, MD: Brookes Publishing.

Wehmeyer, M. L., & Shogren, K. A. (2013). Self-determination: Getting students involved in leadership. In P. Wehman (Ed.), *Life beyond the classroom: Transition strategies for young people with disabilities* (5th ed., pp. 41–68). Baltimore, MD: Brookes Publishing.

Winsor, J. E., Butterworth, J., & Coone, J. (2011). Jobs by 21 Partnership Project: Impact of cross-system collaboration on employment outcome of young adults with disabilities. *Intellectual and Developmental Disabilities, 49*, 274–328. https://doi.org/10.1352/1934-9556-49.4.274.

Workforce innovation and opportunity Act (WIOA), 29 U.S.C. § 3101.(2014).

Yarbrough, D., Getzel, E. E., & Kester, J. (2014). *A topical brief: Expectations of families with young adults with intellectual and developmental disabilities for postsecondary education*. Retrieved from: http://wp.vcu.edu/vcucfi/wp-content/uploads/sites/1763/2012/08/Parent-Expectations-Topical-Brief.pdf.

CHAPTER FOUR

Post-High School Transition for Individuals With Down Syndrome

Marie Moore Channell*,[1] and Susan J. Loveall[§]
*University of Illinois at Urbana-Champaign, Champaign, IL, United States
[§]University of Mississippi, 301 George Hall, University, MS, United States
[1]Corresponding Author: Email: channell@illinois.edu

Contents

International Review of Research in Developmental Disabilities, Volume 54
ISSN 2211-6095
https://doi.org/10.1016/bs.irrdd.2018.07.003

Abstract

As individuals with Down syndrome (DS) are living longer, there is a growing need to support this population across the lifespan. In particular, the transition out of high school marks a critical time point that sets the course for the rest of adulthood, especially for the outcomes of *community-based living, post-secondary education, employment*, and *community engagement*. Little is known about these outcomes in adults with DS, who may experience unique post-school challenges and opportunities relative to those with other intellectual and developmental disabilities. In this paper, we review the state of the literature on post-high school transition outcomes in DS and infuse a phenotypic approach to highlight individual and environmental characteristics associated with these outcomes. We also emphasize current service delivery needs and gaps in the evidence base that must be addressed in order to best support this population during the critical post-high school transition period.

1. INTRODUCTION

Over the last few decades, medical advancements have significantly extended the life expectancy of individuals with Down syndrome (DS), who are now commonly living, on average, into their 60s (Bittles & Glasson, 2004). It has become increasingly important to consider how to best support individuals with DS across the lifespan, including during adulthood. The transition out of high school is a major life event representing a time in which critical decisions are made regarding where to live and how to spend their time, setting the course for the rest of their adult lives. There also are likely unique challenges, needs, and opportunities to succeed during this time period for those with specific phenotypes such as DS (Blacher, Kraemer, & Howell, 2010; Esbensen, Bishop, Seltzer, Greenberg, & Taylor, 2010). However, research on the post-high school transition period within DS is in its infancy. The purpose of this paper is to describe the state of the literature on post-high school transition in DS and to identify directions for future research. Employing the Individuals with Disabilities Education Act (IDEA; 2004) framework, we define transition outcomes in terms of *community-based living, post-secondary education, employment*, and *community engagement*.

Fortunately, societal advancements in disability rights have brought to the forefront the goal of community-based inclusion for individuals with DS and other disabilities (Administration for Community Living, n.d.). That is, these individuals have the basic right to be included and fully integrated into society in all aspects of their daily lives (Americans with Disabilities Act [ADA], 1990). Thus, we must consider how to provide optimal supports to help individuals with DS achieve their goals as they transition out of high school and into community-based settings. Accordingly, this paper will also include characteristics related to transition success in DS, current service delivery needs, and gaps in the evidence base that must be addressed in order to best support this population during this critical transition period.

1.1 What is Transition?

Individuals experience many transitions, or shifts in their environment, throughout the lifespan. In particular, the transition out of high school and into adulthood is one of the biggest rites of passage in modern American culture. For individuals with disabilities such as DS in the United States, this also represents a transition from receiving services through the educational system to receiving community-based services.

To prepare for this transition, at age 14 years individuals in collaboration with their families and educational service providers begin designing a transition plan, a right outlined in IDEA. According to IDEA, the transition plan is an extension of the federally mandated Individualized Education Program (IEP) that is reviewed and implemented annually in American public schools. During transition planning, the school must first conduct assessments and then work with individuals and their families to create annual goals and objectives toward achieving post-high school outcomes. Decisions are made about the individual's long-term goals regarding community-based living, post-secondary education, employment, and community engagement (i.e., the extent to which the individual participates in leisure and recreational activities with others in the community; IDEA, 2004; U.S. Department of Education, 2017). From there, the schools determine appropriate transition services and identify supports to help the individual reach these goals.

Transition plans should be based on each individual's needs and take into account personal strengths, preferences, and interests. When interviewed about their definition of a "good life" and barriers and facilitators to achieving this, young adults with DS who participated in a recent qualitative study reported a desire for more autonomy, especially in independent living and employment domains. Family and community resources were identified as both facilitators and barriers to their desired autonomy and thus quality of life (Scott, Foley, Bourke, Leonard, & Girdler, 2013). Therefore, these areas may be particularly important to individuals with DS as they enter adulthood.

1.2 Achieving Successful Transition to Adulthood

What is considered "successful" transitioning lies in the eye of the beholder. It varies from individual to individual and from family to family. It is also impacted by cultural distinctions, particularly in terms of expectations from the individual's community and family regarding employment, community engagement, role expectations, and social functioning (Blue-Banning, Turnbull, & Pereira, 2002; Geenen, Powers, Vasquez, & Versani, 2003). Because individuals with DS require additional supports from others, there are usually multiple stakeholders involved. Ideally, families and educational service providers will work together to involve the individual in such discussions of what is considered successful transitioning out of high school (IDEA, 2004). In addition to goal setting, individuals with DS and their transition team must identify the appropriate services and training opportunities that will help them achieve their goals (U.S. Department of Education, 2017). Despite this principle, transition planning in practice is widely varied. Therefore, research into the factors that predict successful transitioning and long-term adult outcomes is key to identifying the optimal services and training.

In the early 2000s, the United States Department of Education conducted the National Longitudinal Transition Study-2 (NLTS2, n.d.) to document such experiences of individuals with all types of disabilities and their families from the time they began the transition planning process at age 14 through early adulthood. This survey has provided valuable broad-based information on transitioning and paved the way for other descriptive studies that quantify and qualify transition outcomes and characteristics associated with more positive outcomes. However, these surveys have mixed different known and unknown subgroups (i.e., etiologies) of intellectual and developmental disabilities, making it difficult to track outcomes by etiology. In order to personalize supports during the transition process to meet the needs of individuals with specific types of disabilities such as DS, a more fine-tuned approach to documenting this process is needed. Therefore, taking a phenotypic approach to better understanding the transition process for individuals with DS is an important starting point to supporting these individuals as they enter adulthood.

1.3 Phenotypic Approach

Researchers in the field of intellectual and developmental disabilities have recognized the value of taking a phenotypic approach to understanding how development unfolds across the lifespan for specific etiologies such as

DS (see Karmiloff-Smith et al., 2016), resulting in the description of etiology-specific phenotypes. Here, a phenotype refers to observable characteristics that are more likely to exist in an individual with a particular etiology of disability than in others without the disability (Dykens, 1995).

Key characteristics of the DS phenotype include relative strengths in adaptive skills (i.e., activities of daily living in self-care, community, and communication domains) and social behaviors (Fidler, 2005; Fidler, Most, Booth-LaForce, & Kelly, 2008), some aspects of visual processing (Yang, Conners, & Merrill, 2014), and receptive vocabulary (Abbeduto, Warren, & Conners, 2007; Martin, Klusek, Estigarribia, & Roberts, 2009; McDuffie, Thurman, Channell, & Abbeduto, 2017). These relative strengths are apparent in contrast to difficulties in nonverbal cognitive development (Chapman & Hesketh, 2000) and communication, especially regarding speech intelligibility (Kumin, 1994), expressive language, and grammar (Abbeduto et al., 2007; McDuffie et al., 2017). Aspects of executive functioning, including working memory (Lanfranchi, Jerman, Dal Pont, Alberti, & Vianello, 2010; Loveall, Conners, Tungate, Hahn, & Osso, 2017), are also impaired in this population. Additionally, individuals with DS frequently have difficulties with gross motor development (Winders, 2013) and are at an increased risk for several health concerns (Capone et al., 2018) such as orthopedic problems, vision and hearing issues, seizures, and thyroid dysfunction (Buchanan, 1990; Cohen, 2006; Coleman, 1994; Puri, Ho, & Singh, 2001; Stephen, Dickson, Kindley, Scott, & Charleton, 2007). Importantly, individuals with DS are also at an increased risk of early age-related cognitive declines and early onset Alzheimer's disease (Chapman & Hesketh, 2000; Zigman & Lott, 2007).

The phenotypic approach has also been guided by developmental theories such as the dynamic systems framework (Fidler, Lunkenheimer, & Hahn, 2011) and cascading genetic and environmental effects (Massand & Karmiloff-Smith, 2015). These and other related theories posit that outcomes are the product of interactions among genetic, individual, and environmental processes over time (Granic, 2005; Masten & Cicchetti, 2010; Thelen & Smith, 2006). Thus, applied to DS, the specific genetic influences caused by an extra copy of the 21st chromosome lead to a common phenotype but with inter-individual differences emerging over time that influence and are influenced by aspects of the environment (Fidler et al., 2011).

This approach provides a nice way of considering multiple potential influences on post-high school transition outcomes within DS because it allows for the consideration of complex factors within and across individuals and their environments. For example, two phenotypic language characteristics of DS include poor expressive language and poor speech intelligibility. It is possible that these difficulties may become increasingly apparent in adolescence and young adulthood as the environmental demands of social interaction increase. Ultimately, difficulty communicating with others may negatively impact participation in society, particularly in the areas of community engagement and employment. Further, the premature neurocognitive decline (e.g., working memory and other executive functions) that begins as early as late adolescence for some (Conners, Tungate, Abbeduto, Merrill, & Faught, 2018) and is unique to the DS phenotype (Zigman & Lott, 2007) may also lead to difficulties keeping up with the demands of some work environments. In contrast, the strong social behaviors and relatively strong adaptive skills associated with the DS phenotype may serve as protective factors and lend themselves to more functional skills that result in increased job opportunities and residential independence.

1.3.1 Individual Differences

There is also great inter-individual variation within the DS phenotype, and thus individual difference factors are also important to consider (Karmiloff-Smith et al., 2016). In other words, what is true for most individuals for DS will not be true for every individual with DS. These individual differences can include level of cognitive ability, language and communication skills, adaptive behavior, and psychiatric status (Hodapp, 2007), all of which could impact transition opportunities and needs. Thus, as we identify potential predictors of post-high school outcomes for individuals with DS, both the phenotype and inter-individual differences will be important considerations.

1.3.2 Family

At the environmental level, one especially salient factor relevant to transitioning is the family (Blacher, 2001). For example, parents play an especially large role by identifying post-secondary education/training and employment opportunities and in ensuring that the necessary supports are in place (Brown, Wehmeyer, Webb, & Seabrooks-Blackmore, 2017). Parents of typically developing children often gain a certain amount of independence once their child completes high school and moves out of the family home. However, for parents of an individual with DS, they may actually gain responsibilities once their child transitions out of high school as their child no longer has a structured day of educational experiences and social interactions organized by the school.

On the other hand, research has also documented a "DS advantage", in which parents of children with DS experience greater well-being than parents of children with other intellectual and developmental disabilities (Abbeduto et al., 2004; Corrice & Glidden, 2009; Esbensen & Seltzer, 2011; Stoneman, 2007). These relationships could impact post-high school decisions in terms of level of family involvement. Furthermore, the association between increased maternal age and likelihood of having a child with DS (Martin, Hamilton, Osterman, Curtin, & Mathews, 2015) means that some mothers will be older as their young adult with DS transitions out of high school. This could mean increased financial stability, increased well-being (paired with the "DS advantage"), and other protective factors. However, because these mothers are approaching older adulthood when their child with DS is a young adult, they may find providing informal supports such as coordinating appointments, social outings, and transportation more challenging due to their own declining abilities (Hodapp, Burke, Finley, & Urbano, 2016). Either way, the role that parents and families play during the transition process is crucial for identifying supports and barriers to post-school outcomes for individuals with DS.

1.3.3 Education

Another particularly important environmental consideration is the role of education. For individuals with intellectual disabilities broadly, type of school setting (i.e., inclusive vs. self-contained) is linked to later employment outcomes (Foley et al., 2013). As research has begun to examine the best methods of instruction specifically for individuals with DS (e.g., in the domain of literacy; for discussion see Lemons & Fuchs, 2010), the next step is to assess their impact on long-term outcomes in adults with DS. Thus, the educational environment, including classroom type and instructional programming, is also a crucial consideration as we examine post-high school transition in DS.

2. TRANSITIONING TO ADULTHOOD WITH DOWN SYNDROME: CURRENT OUTCOMES AND POTENTIAL PREDICTORS

Below, we take a phenotypic approach to outline the state of the literature on post-high school transition outcomes for individuals with DS across the categories of community-based living, post-secondary education, employment, and community engagement. Because there is such little research specific to the period of time in which individuals with DS transition from high school (i.e., during their 20s), we broaden our scope to include relevant data more broadly across a wider age range (i.e., throughout adulthood, post-transition) representing long-term adult outcomes. For each outcome, we also highlight potential individual (DS phenotype and individual differences) and environmental (family and education) factors. After reviewing the available research associated with each outcome, we will discuss next steps for the field.

2.1 Community-Based Living

According to McGinley (2002), "housing can be the cornerstone to independence" (p. 83). One's residential setting defines how integrated an individual is within the community (e.g., living in a group home with others who have disabilities vs. living in an apartment complex that houses individuals without disabilities) and the level of supports received (e.g., access to public transportation). Most importantly, having housing options reflects having control over where one lives. For individuals with disabilities, landmark legislation from the 1999 Olmstead United States Supreme Court case made this a legal possibility (Olmstead vs. L. C., 1999). That is, the Supreme Court ruled that an individual's rights under the ADA (1990) include community placements in less restrictive settings. For example, individuals with disabilities are eligible for affordable housing options provided by the government through the United States Department of Housing and Urban Development's Housing Choice Voucher Program, Section 8 (n.d.). Below we outline the recent literature describing community-based living in individuals with DS to determine where we are now.

In the last couple of decades, only a few survey studies have reported on the residential settings of adults with DS in the United States (Esbensen et al., 2010; Stancliffe et al., 2012; Woodman, Mailick, Anderson, & Esbensen, 2014). Although there are still relatively high rates of adults with DS living with relatives (Stancliffe et al., 2012), it appears that over the past 20 years, there has been a trend toward fewer living with their relatives and more living in the community. For example, according to archival data that were collected from a sample of adults with DS of all ages (i.e., 22 years or older) in 1997–98, the vast majority (78%) lived with family (Esbensen et al., 2010). Using data from 2006–08, a large-scale survey conducted by the National Core Indicator across 25 states analyzed the reported residential types in >1000 adults with DS and found that 43% were still living with relatives (Stancliffe et al., 2012). Importantly, this survey represented a subset of adults with DS who *were* receiving state services yet still found a high rate of living with families. Most recently, at the 2010–2011 time point in their longitudinal cohort of adults with DS, Woodman et al. (2014) reported that 35% were residing with relatives. Although the observed trend indicates a decrease in the proportion of adults with DS living with relatives over time, additional findings in Stancliffe's nation-wide study are quite striking. Forty-three percent of adults with DS were still living with relatives, whereas only 28% of individuals with other types of intellectual and developmental disabilities were living with relatives at the same time point (Stancliffe et al., 2012).

The surveys reported above were all conducted in the United States and yielded results similar to that of a large-scale survey ($n = 927$) conducted in 2009 in England and Wales, in which 57% of adults with DS were still living with relatives (Cumella & Heslam, 2014). These findings, however, are substantially different from those of Foley et al. (2014), who reported that 90% of their cohort of adults with DS in Australia were still living with their families. Foley et al.'s sample, however, was much younger (16–30 years old) than those from the United States and the United Kingdom, making it unclear whether the differences observed in the Australian sample were due to services varying across countries and/or age of the sample.

Those adults with DS in the above-mentioned United States-based surveys who were no longer living with relatives varied in terms of level of community integration and independence associated with their residential setting, thus the extent of "community-based living". In Stancliffe et al.'s sample, 23% lived in a group home; 10% lived in an agency apartment and thus were considered to be semi- or fully independent. Woodman et al. (2014) documented similar trends, with 48% of their sample residing in community-based settings; 12% reported living semi- or fully independently. Other residential settings included medical or intermediate care type facilities that tend to serve those who have more complex medical needs (10%, Stancliffe et al., 2012; 5%, Woodman et al., 2014).

Importantly, Cumella and Heslam (2014) included questions in their parent survey regarding satisfaction with their child's current living arrangement. The majority of parents whose children lived in supported housing (i.e., semi-independently in the community) indicated general satisfaction with the supports received, though they also reported informally supplementing these supports. The parents of those who were not in supported housing, most of whom were still living with their families, reported more dissatisfaction with access to formal supports, including an average waiting time of 2.8 years before receiving those supports. This provides evidence of unmet service needs in adults with DS and their families in the United Kingdom. However, we cannot draw any conclusions regarding what proportion of adults with DS and their families are satisfied with their residential arrangements in the United States. This is an important piece of missing data because what is considered a successful transition (in this case, achieving one's ideal residential setting) is defined by each individual and family.

2.1.1 Factors Associated With Community-Based Living

2.1.1.1 Individual level factors

Both age and adaptive functioning emerged as significant correlates of residential status at the 20-year time point of Woodman et al.'s (2014) cohort in the United States; adaptive functioning remained significant even after controlling for age. Those who lived in semi- or fully-independent settings had significantly stronger adaptive skills than those in other settings, and those living with relatives had significantly stronger adaptive skills than those living in nursing homes or hospitals. Although it is possible that living in more independent settings may further strengthen adaptive skills, there is also evidence for a causal relationship in the opposite direction. That is, adaptive behavior from Time 1 predicted community-based living 20 years later. Specifically, those with higher initial levels of adaptive behavior were more likely to live semi- or fully-independently in the community in 20 years (Woodman et al., 2014). Woodman et al. also examined behavior problems and physical health but found no significant patterns of association with residential type. Thus, there is strong evidence for a positive association specifically between adaptive functioning, a predictor at the individual level, and residential independence for adults with DS.

Age also emerged as a significant individual level factor associated with residential type in Stancliffe et al.'s (2012) United States nationwide survey, corroborating Woodman et al.'s (2014) findings. More specifically, in Stancliffe et al.'s sample, those under age 50 were significantly less likely to live independently and more likely to live with relatives than those who were 50 years or older. Visual analysis revealed a steady decline in the proportion of individuals living with family, from 73% in the 18- to 29-year age range to 18% in the 50- to 59-year age range. It should be noted, however, that because there was no measure of adaptive functioning in this sample, the relative contribution of adaptive skills that also can be associated with age is unknown.

2.1.1.2 Environmental level factors

We suspect that the high percentage of individuals with DS who still live with relatives, especially those in the younger age groups, reflects unmet service needs (Cumella & Heslam, 2014), an environmental level factor. This aligns with Woodman et al.'s (2014) conclusions and what is reported in the broader literature on intellectual and developmental disabilities. For example, a report by the Arc FINDS National Survey on intellectual and developmental disabilities in the United States found that only 43% of family caregivers expressed that the current living arrangement for their adult child was ideal; over 40% of family caregivers expressed various unmet support needs related to their relative's current residential arrangement (Anderson, Larson, & Wuorio, 2011). Importantly, the FINDS Survey is one of the only surveys to include both families who are not receiving formal adult services (e.g., Medicaid waiver) in addition to families currently receiving services and thus is more broadly representative of the population. The survey's findings are especially relevant to young adults with DS because of the disproportionately high numbers of young adults living with family in DS relative to other intellectual and developmental disabilities (Stancliffe et al., 2012).

These data are somewhat alarming given the higher maternal age associated with DS (Martin et al., 2015). That is, because mothers of individuals with DS tend to be older, one might expect that the need for additional supports in caring for their adult with DS may come at an earlier age than for families of adults with other intellectual disabilities (Hodapp et al., 2016). However, with evidence to the contrary in terms of reported residential arrangements (i.e., many individuals with DS living with relatives until their 50s), it is possible that there are even greater unmet service needs for families of adults with DS. An additional potential phenotype-specific complication is early cognitive decline and other age-related changes commonly observed in adults with DS by their 40s, if not earlier in life (Torr, Strydom, Patti, & Jokinen, 2010; Zigman, 2013). These likely involve changing service needs such as additional residential supports and healthcare provisions (Hodapp, Perkins, Finley, & Urbano, 2015; Hodapp et al., 2016). Finally, the "DS advantage" noted previously may also partially explain why individuals with DS live at home for longer periods of time.

Parents may feel particularly close to their children with DS and not feel the need for their children to move out as quickly, although future research is needed to explore this possibility.

2.1.2 Summary of Empirical Findings: Community-Based Living

Despite major advancements toward the goal of community-based housing opportunities since the closing of institutions (Lakin, Larson, Salmi, & Webster, 2010), individuals with intellectual and developmental disabilities, including DS, still experience barriers (e.g., long wait lists) to accessing necessary supports such as housing assistance (see McGinley, 2002) and other home- and community-based services (e.g., transportation; healthcare; Anderson et al., 2011). There are still very low numbers of adults with DS considered to be living even semi-independently in the community. Further, individuals with DS are more likely than peers with other intellectual and developmental disabilities to live with parents or other relatives for longer into adulthood rather than moving into more independent settings (Stancliffe et al., 2012). This finding remains despite the observation that across the past 20 years there has been a decrease in the proportion of adults with DS living with family (Esbensen et al., 2010; Stancliffe et al., 2012; Woodman et al., 2014). This pattern, however, should be interpreted with great caution because it is based on only three studies consisting of separate samples (that is, not longitudinal data). Even less is known about current residential types for individuals with DS outside of the United States (see Cumella & Heslam, 2014; Foley et al., 2014). Globally, future work is needed to differentiate types of residential settings and levels of independence in those settings to gain insight into the experiences of adults with DS and their families across the lifespan.

If individuals with DS living with relatives through early and middle adulthood is a reflection of unmet service needs, research should identify what these needs are and why they may be unique to DS. For example, it is possible that alternative residential arrangements supporting the needs and wishes of young adults with DS are not accessible in a timely and financially feasible manner, so families may continue to assume the role of caregivers for a longer period of time, delaying entry into community-based living. Therefore, we also recommend that research identifies the needs and wishes of young adults with DS and their families regarding residential arrangements, similar to what has been completed in the broader population with intellectual and developmental disabilities in the United States (Anderson et al., 2011; Burke & Heller, 2017).

2.2 Post-Secondary Education

Of all the listed post-high school outcomes, there is the greatest lack of research on post-secondary education in DS. What is available suggests that although individuals with DS may seek out some training and education after high school, the nature of that training is very limited. For example, in a sample of 164 young people with DS in Australia, only 17 individuals, or 10%, were attending "training" as their main day occupation (Foley et al., 2014). Training, in this study, included post-secondary education and Technical and Further Education (TAFE) courses. In contrast, a decade or so earlier, also in Australia, more than half ($n = 59$, 54%) of a sample of adults with DS was enrolled in some course of further study, including literacy and numeracy programs, life skills training, work training, and performing arts training programs (Jobling & Cuskelly, 2002). Attendance varied from daily to twice a week and lasted anywhere from 6 weeks to 12 months, thus relatively short-term.

In the United States, the only recent evidence comes from a survey examining employment in adults with DS, in which 12% of the unemployed subsample cited attending a post-secondary education program or other training program as the reason (Kumin & Schoenbrodt, 2016). It remains unknown how many in the broader sample were enrolled in or had completed post-secondary education.

It is quite likely that the paucity of research on post-secondary education in DS reflects the lack of opportunities for individuals with DS to enroll in post-secondary education and achieve this outcome. Current calculations estimate there are 268 college programs for students with intellectual disabilities in the United States (Think College, 2018). Many states have only one such program, and many programs have very limited enrollment ability, often as low as 5–10 students, though the exact number of individuals with DS attending these schools is unknown. The lack of opportunities to attain post-secondary education likely has detrimental effects on acquiring competitive and integrated employment as mandated under the IDEA and the Rehabilitation Act of 1973 (U.S. Department of Education, 2017). Research by Moore and Schelling (2015) on adults with intellectual disabilities is consistent with this explanation; participants who attended post-secondary education programs were more likely to report positive employment outcomes than those who did not attend post-secondary training. This, however, has not yet been examined specifically in DS.

2.2.1 Summary of Empirical Findings: Post-Secondary Education

It is difficult to draw many conclusions regarding post-secondary education in DS, as this is an especially limited area of research. Individuals with DS may seek additional training after high school, but the exact types of training they receive, as well as the benefits of such training, are not yet clear. Whatever the reason, there is an abundant need for more research on post-secondary education outcomes in individuals with DS. We also recommend research to test the hypothesis that not only do a lack of opportunities exist but that they limit access to competitive employment, acting as barriers to achieving post-high school goals for young adults with DS. Ultimately, we hope this research will be used to facilitate the provision of more post-secondary education and technical training opportunities (e.g., University of Alabama's CrossingPoints; Clemson's ClemsonLIFE program). As more individuals with DS enroll in post-secondary education, we also hope that research begins to identify factors leading to positive outcomes in this domain.

2.3 Employment

According to the United States Department of Education, during transition planning, education-based services operating under the IDEA and the Rehabilitation Act of 1973 are required to facilitate post-high school activities that include "competitive integrated employment" for individuals with disabilities (U.S. Department of Education, 2017). "Competitive integrated employment" means that individuals with disabilities should be compensated comparably to those without disabilities (competitive) in an environment that involves interacting with others without disabilities (integrated). Another option is supportive employment, which includes integrated employment but with additional supports provided for those individuals who have more substantial needs (U.S. Department of Education, 2017). However, as we outline below, there seems to be a disconnect between reported goals and the current reality for many individuals with intellectual disabilities, and in particular DS, and their families when it comes to employment.

One recent national survey conducted in the United States reported a 57% paid employment rate across 511 respondents who completed a questionnaire about employment and related activities for individuals with DS (Kumin & Schoenbrodt, 2016). Importantly, this survey included individuals across a wide age range, but it also included some who were still receiving educational services. Out of the 30% who were reported to be unemployed, a subset was still in high school (17%) or in a training program (12%), and thus not necessarily expected to be employed yet. Regardless, a high number of adults remained who were no longer receiving educational services but still reported to be unemployed. Specifically, 41% of those who were unemployed reported that it was not by choice; that is, they were actively seeking a job, did not have adequate transportation, had been laid off, or were fired.

To our knowledge, Kumin and Schoenbrodt's (2016) survey represents the most comprehensive approach to documenting employment related outcomes for individuals with DS in the United States to date. Their findings are also consistent with another recent smaller-scaled study in the United States, which reported 42% of their sample of young adults with DS to be currently employed (Tomaszewski, Fidler, Talapatra, & Riley, 2018). Although it is difficult to compute an aggregate "employment rate" because the situation is much more nuanced (e.g., not distinguishing community-integrated employment from paid sheltered workshops; only reporting percentages of subsamples without raw numbers; etc.), one of the most interpretable and striking statistics is that out of the 57% of Kumin and Schoenbrodt's (2016) sample who were employed, only 13% reported working for 20 h per week or more (3% in full-time employment).

No matter how one divides it, then, employment outcomes vary drastically for individuals with DS, with very few in the United States spending the majority of their weekdays engaged in paid work and even fewer obtaining competitive integrative employment (Kumin & Schoenbrodt, 2016). However, an unusually large portion (42%) was regularly engaged in unpaid volunteer work, another remarkable finding (Kumin & Schoenbrodt, 2016). Outside of the United States, the story of unemployment is similar if not worse (Bertoli et al., 2011; Foley et al., 2014). Although the recent literature reflects improvements over reports from cohorts aging in previous eras in which institutions were still commonplace (e.g., Carr, 2008; Goldstein, 1988; Putnam, Pueschel, & Gorder Holman, 1988), there is still a long way to go to reach the goal of community integration and inclusion related to employment for this population.

2.3.1 Factors Associated With Employment

2.3.1.1 Individual level factors

Again, adaptive functioning may be a key factor, emerging as a strong statistical predictor of employment in a large sample of adults with DS in Australia (Foley et al., 2013). Specifically, those with higher levels of adaptive functioning were more likely to be in the category of 'open employment (defined as community integrated, either competitive or supported) or advanced vocational training' than in the 'sheltered employment or alternatives to employment' category, even after accounting for age, gender, behavior problems, and overall health. This corresponds with findings from Tomaszewski et al. (2018) that the daily living subdomain of adaptive functioning was associated with greater likelihood of being employed in a smaller sample of adults with DS in the United States. Finally, self-involvement in decision-making during transition planning is related to likelihood of "open employment" after adjusting for age, gender, behavior problems, and adaptive functioning. However, because this effect weakened after adjusting for SES, another driving factor at the environmental level may be SES (Foley et al., 2013).

Cognitive predictors of employment are, maybe surprisingly, underrepresented in the literature. In their study, Tomaszewski et al. (2018) identified working memory (not included in Foley et al.'s survey) as a significant correlate of employment status. However, to our knowledge this is the only research tying cognitive abilities to employment in DS. Theoretically, cognitive abilities would predict one's employment capabilities, either directly or indirectly through one's ability to learn relevant job skills. This idea is corroborated in a recent systematic review of employment predictors for individuals with autism spectrum disorder. Out of 17 factors considered, cognitive ability was the only significant predictor consistently tied to work outcomes (Holwerda, van der Klink, Groothaff, & Brouwer, 2012); this finding, however, has yet to be tested within DS.

Due to concerns of early age-related cognitive declines specific to DS, cognition and age represent important avenues for future research. Although there is already some evidence supporting individual differences in employment by age group in DS (Bertoli et al., 2011), caution should be taken when interpreting this finding. It is not clear whether age itself is a factor or whether it simply represents a cohort effect driven by differences in educational practices and training opportunities or even a third variable (e.g., age may also be associated with cognition or adaptive functioning, which impact employment).

2.3.1.2 Environmental level factors

Type of school has also emerged as a significant factor, at least in Australia (Foley et al., 2013). Individuals with DS who attended an "education support unit" (i.e., receiving special education services within an integrated school but not fully mainstreamed) in a private school setting were more likely to be in open employment. However, SES again weakened this relationship. SES likely impacts access to resources, including the educational environment, at least in terms of type of school (e.g., public vs. private) and level of involvement in transition planning. In the Australian education system, both public and private schools are funded by the government; public schools are fully funded (mostly by the state) and private schools vary in their level of government funding (majority funded by the Commonwealth rather than the state) based on need. Special education services are also provided in both public and private school settings (Report on Government Services, 2017). Thus, Foley et al.'s findings may be unique due to the specific structure of Australia's education system. In individuals with disabilities more broadly in the United States educational system, some of the strongest educational predictors of post-school employment are inclusion in general education, vocational education, and work study (Test et al., 2009). These could also be driving factors for individuals with DS, if future research supports this notion.

An association between family-reported quality of life and open employment has also been reported, even after accounting for the confounding factors of adaptive behavior, problem behaviors, and SES (Foley et al., 2014). Furthermore, level of family supports influenced this relationship. Thus, when supported, the family plays an important role in employment outcomes for adults with DS and could potentially mitigate some of the risk factors associated with lower SES mentioned above. Yet to be explored, however, is what kinds of supports families need to in turn support their adult children with DS.

2.3.2 Summary of Empirical Findings: Employment

The IDEA sets "competitive and integrated employment" as the standard for individuals with intellectual and developmental disabilities to the extent possible (i.e., recognizing that some require more substantial accommodations in "supported employment" settings). However, employment rates appear low for individuals with DS, ranging from 42% to 57% in the United States (Kumin & Schoenbrodt, 2016; Tomaszewski et al., 2018), with the overwhelming majority only working part-time. A similar picture has been described in Italy (Bertoli et al., 2011) and Australia (Foley et al., 2013; 2014). Many individuals with DS (42%) instead fill their days with volunteer work (Kumin & Schoenbrodt, 2016). Although the available research points toward overall lower than expected employment rates, there is a lack of nuanced research classifying types of employment, job satisfaction, reasons for unemployment and underemployment, etc. Regardless, the available data indicate that goals set forth by IDEA are not being met for individuals with DS.

Potential individual-level factors are adaptive functioning (Foley et al., 2013; Tomaszewski et al., 2018) and working memory (Tomaszewski et al., 2018). These factors may be good candidates for programs targeting vocational skills. We recommend additional research into the nature of the relationship between these variables and employment outcomes that will more readily inform practice. Additionally, involvement in transition planning by the individual with DS should be recognized as an important factor, and Foley et al.'s (2013) findings serve as initial evidence for a direct link that can be used to advocate for greater involvement, particularly in lower SES environments.

The most salient environmental factors to emerge are family quality of life (Foley et al., 2014)—possibly reflecting the degree to which service needs are met, SES (Foley et al., 2013), and school type (e.g., private school), although this comes from a cohort living in Australia where the structure of the educational system varies from that of the United States. In the United States, inclusion in general education has been found to be predictive of post-school employment in intellectual and developmental disabilities more broadly (Test et al., 2009), but to our knowledge this area is unexplored specifically in DS.

We reiterate the need to consider personal and family goals related to transition outcomes, in this case employment, as documented by current educational policy in the United States (U.S. Department of Education, 2017). By better detailing individual and family goals, outcomes, and unmet service needs through survey research, we can identify current barriers and potential pathways to implementing policy into practice.

2.4 Community Engagement

Community engagement is yet another transition outcome that is integral to achieving optimal quality of life for individuals with disabilities. Drawing from the International Classification of Functioning, Disability, and Health (WHO, 2001) framework of 'participation', community engagement refers to integrated participation and involvement in community-related activities ranging from volunteer and work opportunities (discussed under the separate goal of employment above) to social clubs or organizations and leisure and recreational activities (see Verdonschot, deWitte, Reichrath, Buntinx, &

Curfs, 2009). In order for individuals with disabilities to achieve a high level of community engagement, then, they must be interacting with individuals without disabilities in their daily life.

A very small literature has documented how individuals with DS spend their free time, and an even smaller literature has done so over the past couple of decades, a period of time in which we would expect to observe higher rates of community engagement due to stated efforts to fully integrate individuals with disabilities into communities. One of the most recent studies was conducted by Mihaila et al. (2017) using the Victoria Longitudinal Study activity questionnaire (Jopp & Hertzog, 2007). This measure, previously validated in the typical adult population, was applied to middle-aged adults with DS (ages 35–50 years) to categorize leisure activities as either active (i.e., 'physical', 'social', and 'mentally stimulating' subdomains) or passive (i.e., watching television). Out of all the activities listed, the most commonly endorsed was passive, with 84% reporting they watched television every day. Within the active categories, "social" is perhaps most relevant to community engagement, and 84% reported engaging at least one social activity 2–3 times a week. The most commonly endorsed social activities were visiting with friends/relatives, going out with friends, eating at restaurants, and attending church. Thus, it appears that, with the exception of attending church services, the most frequent community-related activities for middle-aged adults with DS involved interacting with friends and/or relatives. The extent to which these interactions involved individuals without disabilities is unclear. Like-wise, very few individuals reported attending club meetings or organized social events on a regular basis. Out of the remaining categories, recreational sports are also relevant to community engagement; 37% reported participating in this activity on a weekly basis. Again, however, the level of community integration (e.g., community league vs. special league) is not known. Further, with no typically developing comparison group, it is unknown how these results compare to the larger adult population.

Mihaila et al.'s (2017) findings are largely similar to those from slightly older studies, namely Jobling and Cuskelly's (2002) sample and Carr's (2008) longitudinal cohort, who also reported attending church, recreational sports, and visiting friends as relatively frequent leisure/social activities for adults with DS. Although overall club participation was generally higher in Carr's sample than in that of Mihaila et al., when analyzed by type, very few in Carr's study (i.e., 6–12% across age groups) reported ever participating in community-based clubs where they would have the opportunity to interact with other community members in a more integrated setting.

Although we are encouraged that adults with DS are continuing to engage in social activities with friends in the community after high school, the extent to which they interact with individuals without disabilities in integrated settings is unclear. In a large cohort of adults with DS in Italy, a majority reported limited opportunities to interact with others without disabilities, suggesting that there is a need to further support community engagement in adults with DS (Baccichetti, 2007). To our knowledge, no such study has been conducted in the United States from the past couple of decades. We suspect, however, that adults with DS are not as engaged in integrated and community-based leisure activities to the extent expected in modern society.

2.4.1 Factors Associated With Community Engagement

2.4.1.1 Individual level factors

There is virtually no literature directly examining predictors, or even correlates, of community engagement activities of adults with DS. This is likely reflective of the very small literature in recent decades that even touches on descriptions of leisure activities (Carr, 2008; Jobling & Cuskelly, 2002; Mihaila et al., 2017). The most relevant data point to a pattern of characteristics associated with frequency and type of leisure activity in 30–53 year-olds with DS (Mihaila et al., 2017). Controlling for age, gender, physical health, and emotional/behavioral problems, mental age from the Stanford Binet-5 IQ test was positively associated with *social* leisure activities. Time spent with a caregiver was a family-level factor positively associated with *physical* leisure activities. Because the analyses did not differentiate among types of social (e.g., attending church services; visiting with friends/relatives) and physical (e.g., recreational sports; aerobic exercise) activities that could be considered more or less relevant to community participation, we cannot draw conclusions regarding community engagement. However, these findings demonstrate the need for future research on community engagement to include both individual and family level characteristics as potential facilitators to active participation in the community.

2.4.1.2 Environmental level factors

Most relevant to informing practice are those predictors considered malleable. Although further research is required, we suspect that available services within the community, or lack thereof, may play an important environmental role in the extent of community engagement that adults with DS experience. For example, there is some evidence that many leisure activities outside of the home are organized and supervised by community agencies (Jobling & Cuskelly, 2002). However, families tended to initiate these activities for their adult relative with DS. Thus, there may be extra responsibility placed on family members, as evidenced by recent findings that adults with DS are more likely than those with other intellectual disabilities to depend on family members to provide informal supports for recreational activities (Sanderson, Burke, Urbano, Arnold, & Hodapp, 2017).

2.4.2 Summary of Empirical Findings: Community Engagement

Community engagement is an especially difficult outcome variable to define and measure because adults can engage in a wide variety of leisure activities that may or may not involve interacting with others without disabilities in the community. Involvement with others in the community is an important part of adult life. The available research suggests the most common community related activity for individuals with DS is spending time with family and friends (Mihaila et al., 2017). Although promising, this result may also be tied to the large percentage of individuals with DS who live with relatives, as the available research does not differentiate the extent of integration during community related activities (e.g., dining out with friends with and without disabilities vs. with relatives). Interpersonal relationships (e.g., reciprocal friendships), then, may be the key to increasing community participation for individuals with DS, although additional research is needed to support this empirically.

At the environmental level, two potential predictors of the extent to which adults with DS are involved in recreational activities in the community are family support (Jobling & Cuskelly, 2002) and community services (i.e., access to transportation; organizing and coordinating activities; Esbensen et al., 2010). Again, the family seems to be carrying a substantial amount of the responsibility, particularly for adults with DS relative to other disabilities (Sanderson et al., 2017). Because recreational services and transportation services have been identified as two significant predictors of broad metrics of independence in adults with DS specifically (Esbensen et al., 2010), such services may play a particularly salient role in increasing opportunities for community engagement in this population. Future research should include these variables, as they are particularly amenable to change and, if optimally implemented into practice, would reduce familial responsibilities and increase opportunities for community integration and participation.

3. CONCLUSIONS AND FUTURE DIRECTIONS

With the drastic increase in the life expectancy of individuals with DS over the past 50 years (Bittles & Glasson, 2004), they will now spend the majority of their lives in adulthood. There is a critical need, therefore, to support these individuals as they transition out of high school and to help them achieve their ideal post-school goals. The first step towards accomplishing this is to identify both barriers and facilitators of post-high school outcomes for this population. This should include a phenotypic approach to understand how aspects of the DS phenotype interact with environmental factors over time to impact the independent living outcomes achieved in adulthood. The purpose of this paper was to document post-high school outcomes for individuals with DS in the areas of *community-based living*, *post-secondary education*, *employment*, and *community engagement*, and to identify individual and environmental characteristics associated with each outcome.

In reviewing the literature, one of the first and most consistent themes to emerge was that there is not enough research describing any post-school outcomes in young adults with DS, even in the United States. There is a global need for more research to document outcomes in different countries, across which educational systems and community services may vary. What is currently available spans wide age ranges, seldomly distinguishes different components of the same outcome (e.g., unemployed and seeking employment vs. unemployed but in a training program; employed part-time and volunteering vs. employed full-time; living with relatives and satisfied vs. living with relatives but seeking alternative arrangements; etc.), and rarely considers predictors of each outcome. As a result, a nuanced understanding of how individual differences could lead to differential outcomes is largely uncharted territory.

Some simple additions to future research include reporting both numbers and percentages of individuals in subcategories (e.g., by age group, number of paid hours per week, etc.) and clearly operationalizing outcome variables. This will allow results to be more readily compared and combined across studies and countries to understand the population more broadly and to cast a wider net regarding the types of outcomes that are studied. Additionally, because documentation of changes in these outcomes over time provides valuable information, future endeavors should also begin tracking potential predictors of post-high school outcomes earlier (i.e., during high school) in order to identify pathways for supporting these individuals while they are still planning their transition.

3.1 Post-High School Outcomes

Despite its limitations, the available research has enabled us to begin documenting post-high school outcomes for adults with DS as a first step towards advancing the field. In the domain of community-based living, adults with DS are living with their families more often and for longer periods of time than adults with intellectual and developmental disabilities of other etiologies (Stancliffe et al., 2012). The reason for this, however, is not yet clear. Moving forward, it will be important to document the perspectives of both individuals with DS and their families to better understand their needs and wishes surrounding community-based living and how their perspectives may change over time.

The available research also indicates extremely limited opportunities for post-secondary education and training for individuals with intellectual disabilities broadly, including those with DS (Think College, 2018). Increasing access to such opportunities would likely lead to greater independence in all areas of adulthood. For example, additional training that focuses on functional skills required to live more independently during adulthood could increase opportunities for community-based living. Like-wise, technical and/or vocational training should lead to more competitive employment (see Moore & Schelling, 2015), which could also facilitate housing opportunities. Future research should also specify which post-secondary education/training opportunities lead to achievement of other post-school outcomes in this population.

In terms of community engagement, there is a dearth of evidence regarding the nature and frequency of recreational activities in community-based, integrated settings for individuals with DS. Drawing from a theoretical framework of social inclusion for individuals with intellectual and developmental disabilities, community participation and interpersonal relationships are key pieces to community engagement (Simplican, Leader, Kosciulek, & Leahy, 2015); however, both of these areas may be limited for adults with DS (Mihaila et al., 2017). Many of the leisure activities reported are ambiguous as to level of community integration. Relevant to interpersonal relationships, many reports of social activities involve outings with relatives and thus may be tied to the high number of individuals with DS who live with relatives and not reflective of reciprocal relationships with peers (see Baccichetti, 2007). Reciprocal friendships could play an essential role in community participation for individuals with DS, especially those who have recently transitioned out of high school and lost structured opportunities to interact with peers (see Scott et al., 2013), and future research should examine this possibility. Finally, there remains a need to identify the individual and family supports required for optimal community participation (e.g., coordinating activities; access to transportation; etc.) to reveal ways that communities can improve services for this population after high school.

3.2 Factors Associated With Post-High School Outcomes

Another emerging theme from the extant literature is that adaptive behaviors may be particularly relevant to post-school outcomes in DS (Foley et al., 2013; Tomaszewski et al., 2018; Woodman et al., 2014). Collectively, adaptive behaviors promote independence and thus are related to quality of life throughout the lifespan. This may be particularly relevant in adulthood, a time in which greater expectations are placed on the individual to function independently. Phenotypic research on DS indicates that adaptive functioning may be a strength in individuals with DS, at least relative to other intellectual and developmental disabilities (Esbensen et al., 2010; Zigman, Schupf, Urv, Zigman, & Silverman, 2002). This research, however, also points to loss in adaptive skills with age in DS (Esbensen, Seltzer, & Krauss, 2008; Lin et al., 2013; Maaskant et al., 1996; Matthews et al., 2018), although it is not clear whether this loss is specific to individuals with DS or characteristic of intellectual and developmental disabilities more broadly.

The specific skills needed to exhibit adaptive functioning (e.g., self-care; vocational; etc.) vary based on context and the degree of expectations placed on an individual by the surrounding community (Tassé, 2013). Thus, future work should consider an individual's environmental supports and demands while investigating the link between different types of adaptive skills and various post-school outcomes in DS. For example, because working memory, an important skill for goal-directed behaviors, is an area of difficulty for many individuals with DS (Lanfranchi et al., 2010; Loveall et al., 2017), one direction would be to explore the role of working memory in outcomes such as vocational training and employment (Tomaszewski et al., 2018). Similarly, the role of language and communication should be considered because this is another area of relative weakness in DS (Abbeduto et al., 2007; McDuffie et al., 2017) and amenable to intervention. In fact, there is preliminary evidence that receiving speech-language services in adulthood predicts broad levels of transition independence in adults with

DS, a finding that was unique to DS relative to other developmental disabilities (Esbensen et al., 2010). Therefore, a stronger understanding of the DS phenotype, individual differences, and their impact on post-school outcomes will help specify targets for interventions to support long-term success in adulthood.

Considering environmental influences, another theme to emerge was the large role family members play in the lives of individuals with DS after high school, even relative to other intellectual and developmental disabilities (Hodapp et al., 2015). Not only do individuals with DS live with family longer into adulthood (Cumella & Heslam, 2014; Foley et al., 2014; Stancliffe et al., 2012; Woodman et al., 2014), but family members also bear a majority of the responsibility in other areas, including finding post-secondary education and employment opportunities. Regarding community engagement, family members are often the ones with whom adults with DS spend their leisure time and also tend to coordinate participation in community-based recreational activities (Sanderson et al., 2017). Thus, we recommend that research specifically focuses on how families support post-high school transition for their relative with DS. This work should also lead to the identification of different types of unmet service needs and strategies for improving service delivery for families at the community level. These services will be even more critical for individuals with DS who do not have living relatives to provide supplemental informal supports.

Education represents another important environmental consideration. To our knowledge, none of the studies describing adult independent living outcomes in DS has specifically linked post-school outcomes to prior educational settings/programs in the United States, and only one has alluded to it elsewhere (i.e., Foley et al., 2013). Thus, there is a critical need for research to determine the educational supports that lead to individuals with DS achieving post-secondary goals. Because in the United States, inclusion in the general education classroom, paid employment/work experience during high school, work-study, transition program, and vocational education predict post-school outcomes for individuals with intellectual and developmental disabilities (Test et al., 2009), we recommend that research prioritize studying these factors in individuals with DS. We also do not yet have strong evidence describing what is happening during transition planning in relation to post-school outcomes in DS; again, the educational factors mentioned above represent strong starting points.

3.3 Additional Future Directions

An avenue for future research that did not surface in this review but is important to consider moving forward is the association between post-high school outcomes and mental health in DS. Lower rates of mental health problems have been reported for individuals with DS compared to other etiologies of intellectual disability, leading some to consider the possibility of a genetic protective factor (Mantry et al., 2008; Morgan, Leonard, Bourke, & Jablensky, 2008). However, the onset of mental health problems, particularly withdrawal and depression, has been observed in some adolescents and young adults with DS (Dykens, Shah, Sagun, Beck, & King, 2002). Because environmental factors may play a large role in these cases (Mallardo, Cuskelly, White, & Jobling, 2014), the transition out of high school and away from structured days involving education and peer interaction may be a particularly vulnerable time for these young adults. We recommend that future endeavors work to determine how adult outcomes may impact mental health in DS and vice versa.

Finally, a very important consideration not yet represented in most cohort-based studies (i.e., beyond case study descriptions) is satisfaction regarding community-based living, employment, post-secondary education, and community engagement in DS. For example, what proportion of individuals with DS and their families are satisfied with their current activities in each of these domains (see Cumella & Heslam, 2014)? What are their goals and wishes, and how well are they being supported throughout adulthood? This is an especially important piece of missing data because transition "success" is defined by each individual within the broader context of familial and cultural values.

3.4 Conclusion

The good news is that there has been a recent increase in the literature on post-school outcomes in DS (e.g., Cumella & Heslam, 2014; Foley et al., 2014, 2013; Kumin & Schoenbrodt, 2016; Mihaila et al., 2017; Tomaszewski et al., 2018; Woodman et al., 2014), and we are confident that more evidence is on the horizon using data from these cohort-based investigations. The critical next step will be to identify predictors of successful transition outcomes at the individual, family, and educational levels. This will provide researchers, educators, and other community service providers with multiple potential routes for intervention to better support long-term outcomes for adults with DS and their families.

REFERENCES

Abbeduto, L., Seltzer, M. M., Shattuck, P., Krauss, M. W., Orsmond, G., & Murphy, M. M. (2004). Psychological well-being and coping in mothers of youths with autism, Down syndrome, or fragile X syndrome. *American Journal on Mental Retardation, 109*(3), 237–254.

Abbeduto, L., Warren, S. F., & Conners, F. A. (2007). Language development in Down syndrome: From the prelinguistic period to the acquisition of literacy. *Mental Retardation and Developmental Disabilities Research Reviews, 13*, 247–261.

Administration for Community Living, n.d. Retrieved from: https://www.acl.gov/about-acl.

Americans with disabilities Act of 1990, pub. L. No. 101-336, 104 stat. 328.(1990).

Anderson, L. L., Larson, S. A., & Wuorio, A. (2011). *2010 FINDS National survey technical report part 1: Family caregiver survey*. Minneapolis: University of Minnesota, Research and Training Center on Community Living.

Baccichetti, C. (2007). Quality of life. In J. Rondal, & A. Rasore-Quartino (Eds.), *Therapies and rehabilitation in Down syndrome* (pp. 195–205). New York: John Wiley & Sons, Ltd.

Bertoli, M., Biasini, G., Calignano, M. T., Celani, G., De Grossi, G., Digilio, M. C., … Zuccalà, G. (2011). Needs and challenges of daily life for people with Down syndrome residing in the city of Rome, Italy. *Journal of Intellectual Disability Research: JIDR, 55*(8), 801–820.

Bittles, A. H., & Glasson, E. J. (2004). Clinical, social, and ethical implications of changing life expectancy in Down syndrome. *Developmental Medicine and Child Neurology, 46*, 282–286.

Blacher, J. (2001). Transition to adulthood: Mental retardation, families, and culture. *American Journal on Mental Retardation, 106*, 173–188.

Blacher, J., Kraemer, B., & Howell, E. (2010). Family expectations and transition experiences for young adults with severe disabilities: Does syndrome matter? *Advances in Mental Health and Learning Disabilities, 4*(1), 3–16.

Blue-Banning, M., Turnbull, A. P., & Pereira, L. (2002). Hispanic youth/young adults with disabilities: Parents' visions for the future. *Research and Practice for Persons with Severe Disabilities, 27*(3), 204–219.

Brown, I., Wehmeyer, M. L., Webb, W., & Seabrooks-Blackmore, J. (2017). The transition from school to adult life. In M. L. Wehmeyer, I. Brown, M. Percey, K. A. Shogren, & W. L. A. Fung (Eds.), *A comprehensive guide to intellectual and developmental disabilities* (2nd ed., pp. 541–555). Baltimore, MD: Brookes Publishing.

Buchanan, L. H. (1990). Early onset of presbyacusias in Down syndrome. *Scandinavian Audiology, 19*(2), 103–110.

Burke, M. M., & Heller, T. (2017). Disparities in unmet service needs among adults with intellectual and other developmental disabilities. *Journal of Applied Research in Intellectual Disabilities, 30*, 898–910.

Capone, G. T., Chicoine, B., Bulova, P., Stephens, M., Hart, S., Crissman, B., … Down Syndrome Medical Interest Group DSMIG-USA Adult Health Care Workgroup. (2018). Co-occurring medical conditions in adults with down syndrome: A systematic review toward the development of health care guidelines. *American Journal of Medical Genetics, A, 176*(1), 116–133.

Carr, J. (2008). The everyday life of adults with Down syndrome. *Journal of Applied Research in Intellectual Disabilities, 21*(5), 389–397.

Chapman, R. S., & Hesketh, L. J. (2000). Behavioral phenotype of individuals with Down syndrome. *Mental Retardation and Developmental Disabilities Research Reviews, 6*, 84–95.

Cohen, W. I. (2006). Current dilemmas in Down syndrome clinical care: Celiac disease, thyroid disorders, and atlanto-axial instability. *American Journal of Medical Genetics, C, 142*, 141–148.

Coleman, M. (1994). Thyroid dysfunction in down syndrome: A review. *Down Syndrome: Research and Practice, 2*(3), 112–115.

Conners, F. A., Tungate, A. S., Abbeduto, L., Merrill, E. C., & Faught, G. G. (2018). Growth and decline in language and phonological memory over two years among adolescents with Down syndrome. *American Journal on Intellectual and Developmental Disabilities, 123*, 103–118.

Corrice, A. M., & Glidden, L. M. (2009). The Down syndrome advantage: Fact or fiction? *American Journal on Intellectual and Developmental Disabilities, 114*(4), 254–268.

Cumella, S., & Heslam, S. (2014). Supported housing for people with Down's syndrome. *British Journal of Learning Disabilities, 42*, 251–256.

Dykens, E. M. (1995). Measuring behavioral phenotypes: Provocations from the "new genetics". *American Journal on Mental Retardation, 99*(5), 522–532.

Dykens, E. M., Shah, B., Sagun, J., Beck, T., & King, B. H. (2002). Maladaptive behaviour in children and adolescents with Down's syndrome. *Journal of Intellectual Disability Research: JIDR, 46*(6), 484–492.

Esbensen, A. J., Bishop, S., Seltzer, M. M., Greenberg, J. S., & Taylor, J. L. (2010). Comparisons between individuals with autism spectrum disorders and individuals with Down syndrome in adulthood. *American Journal on Intellectual and Developmental Disabilities, 115*(4), 277–290.

Esbensen, A. J., & Seltzer, M. M. (2011). Accounting for the "Down syndrome advantage". *American Journal on Intellectual and Developmental Disabilities, 116*(1), 3–15.

Esbensen, A. J., Seltzer, M. M., & Krauss, M. W. (2008). Stability and change in health, functional abilities and behavior problems among adults with and without Down syndrome. *American Journal on Mental Retardation, 113*, 263–277.

Fidler, D. J. (2005). The emerging Down syndrome behavioral phenotype in early childhood. *Infants & Young Children, 18*, 86–103.

Fidler, D. J., Lunkenheimer, E., & Hahn, L. (2011). Emerging behavioral phenotypes and dynamic systems theory. In *International review of research in developmental disabilities* (Vol. 40, pp. 17–42). Academic Press.

Fidler, D. J., Most, D. E., Booth-LaForce, C., & Kelly, J. F. (2008). Emerging social strengths in young children with Down syndrome. *Infants & Young Children, 21*(3), 207–220.

Foley, K.-R., Girdler, S., Downs, J., Jacoby, P., Bourke, J., Lennox, N., … Leonard, H. (2014). Relationship between family quality of life and day occupations of young people with Down syndrome. *Social Psychiatry and Psychiatric Epidemiology, 49*, 1455–1465.

Foley, K.-R., Jacoby, P., Girdler, S., Bourke, J., Pikora, T., Lennox, N., … Leonard, H. (2013). Functioning and post-school transition outcomes for young people with Down syndrome. *Child: Care, Health and Development, 39*(6), 789–800.

Geenen, S., Powers, L., Vasquez, A. L., & Bersani, H. (2003). Understanding and promoting the transition of minority adolescents. *Career Development for Exceptional Individuals, 26*(1), 27–46.

Goldstein, H. (1988). Living conditions of an adult population with Down's syndrome. *Research in Developmental Disabilities, 9*(2), 123–134.

Granic, I. (2005). Timing is everything: Developmental psychopathology from a dynamic systems perspective. *Developmental Review, 25*, 386–407. https://doi.org/10.1016/j.dr.2005.10.005.

Hodapp, R. M. (2007). Families of persons with Down syndrome: New perspectives, findings, and research and service needs. *Mental Retardation and Developmental Disabilities Research Reviews, 13*, 279–287.

Hodapp, R. M., Burke, M. M., Finley, C. I., & Urbano, R. C. (2016). Family caregiving of aging adults with Down syndrome. *Journal of Policy and Practice in Intellectual Disabilities, 13*, 181–189.

Hodapp, R. M., Perkins, A. M., Finley, C. I., & Urbano, R. C. (2015). Growing old together: Similarities/differences in families of adults with and without Down syndrome. In *International review of research in developmental disabilities* (Vol. 49, pp. 151–189). Academic Press.

Holwerda, A., van der Klink, J. J. L., Groothoff, J. W., & Brouwer, S. (2012). Predictors for work participation for individuals with an autism spectrum disorder: A systematic review. *Journal of Occupational Rehabilitation, 22*, 333–352.

Individuals with disabilities education Act, 20 U.S.C. § 1400.(2004).

Jobling, A., & Cuskelly, M. (2002). Life styles of adults with down syndrome living at home. In M. Cuskelly, A. Jobling, & S. Buckley (Eds.), *Down syndrome across the life span* (pp. 109–120). Philadelphia: Whurr Publishers.

Jopp, D. S., & Hertzog, C. (2007). Activities, self-referent memory beliefs, and cognitive performance: Evidence for direct and mediated relations. *Psychology and Aging, 22*(4), 811–825.

Karmiloff-Smith, A., Al-Janabi, T., D'Souza, H., Groet, J., Massand, E., Mok, K., … Strydom, A. (2016). The importance of understanding individual differences in Down syndrome. *F1000Research, 5*, F1000. Faculty Rev–389.

Kumin, L. (1994). Intelligibility of speech in children with Down syndrome in natural settings: Parents' perspective. *Perceptual & Motor Skills, 78*(1), 307–313.

Kumin, L., & Schoenbrodt, L. (2016). Employment in adults with Down syndrome in the United States: Results from a national survey. *Journal of Applied Research in Intellectual Disabilities, 29*(4), 330–345.

Lakin, K., Larson, S., Salmi, P., & Webster, A. (2010). *Residential services for persons with developmental disabilities: Status and trends through 2009.* Research and Training Center on Community Living Institute on Community Integration/UCEDD, College of Education and Human Development, University of Minnesota. http://rtc.umn.edu/docs/risp2009.pdf.

Lanfranchi, S., Jerman, O., Dal Pont, E., Alberti, A., & Vianello, R. (2010). Executive function in adolescents with Down syndrome. *Journal of Intellectual Disability Research: JIDR, 54*(4), 308–319.

Lemons, C. J., & Fuchs, D. (2010). Phonological awareness of children with Down syndrome: Its role in learning to read and the effectiveness of related interventions. *Research in Developmental Disabilities, 31*, 316–330.

Lin, L., Hsia, Y., Hsu, S., Loh, C., Wu, C., & Lin, J. (2013). Caregivers' reported functional limitations in activities of daily living among middle-aged adults with intellectual disabilities. *Research in Developmental Disabilities, 34*(12), 4559–4564.

Loveall, S. J., Conners, F. A., Tungate, A. S., Hahn, L. J., & Osso, T. D. (2017). A cross-sectional analysis of executive function in Down syndrome from 2 to 35 years. *Journal of Intellectual Disability Research: JIDR, 61*, 877–887. https://doi.org/10.1111/jir.12396.

Maaskant, M. A., van den Akker, M., Kessels, A. G. H., Haveman, M. J., van Schrojenstein Lantman-de Valk, H. M. J., & Urlings, H. F. J. (1996). Care dependence and activities of daily living in relation to ageing: Results of a longitudinal study. *Journal of Intellectual Disability Research: JIDR, 40*, 535–543.

Mallardo, M., Cuskelly, M., White, P., & Jobling, A. (2014). Mental health problems in adults with Down syndrome and their association with life circumstances. *Journal of Mental Health Research in Intellectual Disabilities, 7*, 229–245.

Mantry, D., Cooper, S.-A., Smiley, E., Morrison, J., Allan, L., Williamson, A., … Jackson, A. (2008). The prevalence and incidence of mental ill-health in adults with Down syndrome. *Journal of Intellectual Disability Research: JIDR, 52*, 141–155.

Martin, J., Hamilton, B., Osterman, M., Curtin, M., & Mathews, M. (2015). Births: Final data for 2013 internet tables. In *National vital statistics reports* (Vol. 1 Suppl.). Retrieved from: www.cdc.gov/nchs/data/nvsr/nvsr64/nvsr64_01_tables.pdf.

Martin, G. E., Klusek, J., Estigarribia, B., & Roberts, J. E. (2009). Language characteristics of individuals with Down syndrome. *Topics in Language Disorders, 29*(2), 112–132. https://doi.org/10.1097/TLD.0b013e3181a71fe1.

Massand, E., & Karmiloff-Smith, A. (2015). Cascading genetic and environmental effects on development: Implications for intervention. In K. J. Mitchell (Ed.), *The genetics of neurodevelopmental disorders (275–288)*. Hoboken, NJ: John Wiley & Sons.

Masten, A. S., & Cicchetti, D. (2010). Developmental cascades. *Development and Psychopathology, 22*(3), 491–495.

Matthews, T. J., Allain, D. C., Matthews, A. L., Mitchell, A., Santoro, S. L., & Cohen, L. (2018). An assessment of health, social, communication, and daily living skills of adults with Down syndrome. *American Journal of Medical Genetics*. advanced online publication.

McDuffie, A., Thurman, A. J., Channell, M. M., & Abbeduto, L. (2017). Language disorders in children with intellectual disability of genetic origin. In R. Schwartz (Ed.), *Handbook of child language disorders* (2nd ed., pp. 52–81). New York: Taylor & Francis.

McGinley, K. H. (2002). Playing the housing "game": People with Down syndrome and their families can have more control when it comes to housing. In W. I. Cohen, L. Nadel, & M. E. Madnick (Eds.), *Down syndrome: Visions for the 21st century* (pp. 83–103). New York: Wiley-Liss, Inc.

Mihaila, L., Hartley, S. L., Handen, B. L., Bulova, P. D., Tumuluru, R. V., Devenny, D. A., … Christian, B. T. (2017). Leisure activity and caregiver involvement in middle-aged and older adults with Down syndrome. *Intellectual and Developmental Disabilities, 55*(2), 97–109.

Moore, E. J., & Schelling, A. (2015). Postsecondary inclusion for individuals with an intellectual disability and its effects on employment. *Journal of Intellectual Disabilities, 19*(2), 130–148.

Morgan, V. A., Leonard, H., Bourke, J., & Jablensky, A. (2008). Intellectual disability co-occurring with and other psychiatric illness: Population-based study. *British Journal of Psychiatry, 193*, 364–372. https://doi.org/10.1192/bjp.bp.107.044461.

NLTS2, n.d. Retrieved from: https://nlts2.sri.com.

Olmstead vs. L. C., 527 U.S. 581 (1999).

Puri, B. K., Ho, K. W., & Singh, I. (2001). Age of seizure onset in adults with Down's syndrome. *International Journal of Clinical Practice, 55*(7), 442–444.

Putnam, J. W., Pueschel, S. M., & Gorder Holman, J. (1988). Community activities of youths and adults with Down syndrome. *British Journal of Mental Subnormality, 34*(1), 47–53.

Report on Government Services. (2017). *School education, volume B, Chapter 4*. Retrieved from: https://www.pc.gov.au/research/ongoing/report-on-government-services/2017/child-care-education-and-training/school-education/rogs-2017-volumeb-chapter4.pdf.

Sanderson, K. A., Burke, M. M., Urbano, R. C., Arnold, C. K., & Hodapp, R. M. (2017). Who helps? Characteristics and correlates of informal supporters to adults with disabilities. *American Journal on Intellectual and Developmental Disabilities, 122*, 492–510.

Scott, M., Foley, K.-R., Bourke, J., Leonard, H., & Girdler, S. (2013). "I have a good life": The meaning of well-being from the perspective of young adults with Down syndrome. *Disability & Rehabilitation, 36*(15), 1464–5165.

Simplican, S. C., Leader, G., Kosciulek, J., & Leahy, M. (2015). Defining social inclusion of people with intellectual and developmental disabilities: An ecological model of social networks and community participation. *Research in Developmental Disabilities, 38*, 18–29.

Stancliffe, R. J., Lakin, K. C., Larson, S. A., Engler, J., Taub, S., Fortune, J., & Bershadsky, J. (2012). Demographic characteristics, health conditions, and residential service use in adults with Down syndrome in 25 U.S. states. *Intellectual and Developmental Disabilities, 50*, 92–108.

Stephen, E., Dickson, J., Kindley, A. D., Scott, C. C., & Charleton, P. M. (2007). Surveillance of vision and ocular disorders in children with Down syndrome. *Developmental Medicine and Child Neurology, 49*, 513–515.

Stoneman, Z. (2007). Examining the Down syndrome advantage: Mothers and fathers of young children with disabilities. *Journal of Intellectual Disability Research: JIDR, 51*(12), 1006–1017.

Tassé, M. J. (2013). Adaptive behavior. In M. L. Wehmeyer (Ed.), *The oxford handbook of positive psychology and disability* (pp. 105–115). New York: Oxford University Press.

Test, D. W., Mazzotti, V. L., Mustian, A. L., Fowler, C. H., Kortering, L., & Kohler, P. (2009). Evidence-based secondary transition predictors for improving postschool outcomes for students with disabilities. *Career Development for Exceptional Individuals, 32*, 160–181.

Thelen, E., & Smith, L. B. (2006). Dynamic systems theories. In R. M. Lerner, & W. Damon (Eds.), *Handbook of child psychology: Volume 1, Theoretical models of human development* (6th ed., pp. 258–312). Hoboken, NJ: John Wiley & Sons, Inc.

Think College. (2018). *College search.* Available from: https://thinkcollege.net/college-search.

Tomaszewski, B., Fidler, D., Talapatra, D., & Riley, K. (2018). Adaptive behaviour, executive function and employment in adults with Down syndrome. *Journal of Intellectual Disability Research: JIDR, 62*(1), 41–52.

Torr, J., Strydom, A., Patti, P., & Jokinen, N. (2010). Aging in down syndrome: Morbidity and mortality. *Journal of Policy and Practice in Intellectual Disabilities, 7*, 70–81.

U.S. Department of Education (Department), Office of Special Education and Rehabilitative Services. (2017). *A transition guide to postsecondary education and employment for students and youth with disabilities.* Washington, D.C.

United States Department of Housing and Urban Development's Housing Choice Voucher Program, Section 8 (n.d.). Retrieved from: https://www.hud.gov/program_offices/housing/mfh/grants/section811ptl.

Verdonschot, M. M. L., deWitte, L. P., Reichrath, E., Buntinx, W. H. E., & Curfs, L. M. G. (2009). Community participation of people with an intellectual disability: A review of empirical findings. *Journal of Intellectual Disability Research: JIDR, 53*, 303–318.

Winders, P. C. (2013). *Gross motor skills for children with Down syndrome: A guide for parents and professionals.* Bethesda, MD: Woodbine House.

Woodman, A. C., Mailick, M. R., Anderson, K. A., & Esbensen, A. J. (2014). Residential transitions among adults with intellectual disability across 20 years. *American Journal on Intellectual and Developmental Disabilities, 119*(6), 496–515. https://doi.org/10.1352/1944-7558-119.6.496.

World Health Organization (WHO). (2001). *International classification of functioning, disability and health.* Geneva: WHO.

Yang, Y., Conners, F. A., & Merrill, E. C. (2014). Visuo-spatial ability in individuals with Down syndrome: Is it really a strength? *Research in Developmental Disabilities, 35*(7), 1473–1500.

Zigman, W. B. (2013). A typical aging in Down syndrome. *Developmental Disabilities and Research Reviews, 18*, 51–67.

Zigman, W. B., & Lott, I. T. (2007). Alzheimer's disease in Down syndrome: Neurobiology and risk. *Mental Retardation and Developmental Disabilities Research Reviews, 13*, 237–246.

Zigman, W. B., Schupf, N., Urv, T., Zigman, A., & Silverman, W. (2002). Incidence and temporal patterns of adaptive behavior change in adults with mental retardation. *American Journal on Mental Retardation, 107*, 161–174.

CHAPTER FIVE

A Review of Supports and Services for Adults With Intellectual and Developmental Disabilities (IDD) and Their Families in the United States: Past and Present Contexts Impacting Future Research, Practice and Policy

Meghan M. Burke[*,1], **Amie Lulinski**[§], **Jennifer Jones**[¶] **and Kami Gallus**[¶]

[*]University of Illinois at Urbana-Champaign, Champaign, IL, United States
[§]Coleman Institute for Cognitive Disabilities, Boulder, CO, United States
[¶]Oklahoma State University, Stillwater, OK, United States
[1]Corresponding Author: Email: meghanbm@illinois.edu

Contents

International Review of Research in Developmental Disabilities, Volume 54
ISSN 2211-6095
https://doi.org/10.1016/bs.irrdd.2018.07.005

Abstract

Given the important roles of family caregivers and the likelihood that individuals with IDD will live in their family homes into adulthood, it is crucial to examine adult service delivery systems within the context of families of individuals with IDD. In this manuscript, we aim to describe the adult service delivery system, specifically with respect to HCBS Medicaid waiver in the United States, and its relation to the contexts and implications of family caregivers for adults with IDD. We begin by providing a history of adult services; then, we shift our focus to community-based support. Next, we discuss the theoretical framework, Family Systems Theory. Then, we describe the contexts and implications of family caregivers. We conclude with directions for future research, practice, and policy. Because this manuscript highlights the complicated nature of adult services, we provide a description and list of the relevant acronyms in Table 1.

In 2016, there were an estimated 7.37 million individuals with intellectual and developmental disabilities (IDD) in the United States (Larson et al., 2018). Because of the increasing lifespans of individuals with IDD, they are beginning to outlive their parents for the first time. Thus, long-term care falls on family members. Indeed, there are almost 43.5 million informal caregivers in the United States (National Alliance for Caregiving, 2015). These caregivers have an economic value ranging from $375 to 470 billion (Reinhard, Feinberg, Choula, & Houser, 2015). With respect to caregivers of individuals with IDD specifically, parents continue to care for their offspring with IDD (Braddock et al., 2015); 71% of individuals with IDD receive support from a family caregiver (Braddock, Hemp, Tanis, Wu, & Haffer, 2017).

To support families of individuals with IDD, especially adults, the federal government funds long-term supports and services (LTSS) through state IDD agencies (Anderson, Larson, Kardell, Taylor, Hallas-Muchow, Eschenbacher, Hewitt, Sowers, & Bourne, 2018). LTSS can include a variety of supports or services for individuals with disabilities. For example, LTSS may include assistance with activities of daily living, day programs, residential programs, and care coordination. Currently, approximately 30% (1.4 million) of individuals with IDD receive LTSS (Anderson et al., 2018).

Table 1 List and Description of Acronyms

Acronym	Term	Definition
IDD	Intellectual and developmental disability	Individuals with an intellectual disability and/or developmental disability
LTSS	Long-term supports and services	Supports or services provided by the government to an individual with IDD
ICF	Intermediate Care Facility	A residential option for individuals with IDD
HCBS	Home and Community-Based Services	A waiver to promote home and community-based services to individuals with IDD
FMAP	Federal Medical Assistance Percentage	A formulate based on state per capita personal income to determine Medicaid reimbursement
ADA	Americans with Disabilities Act	A federal act prohibiting discrimination of individuals with disabilities and requiring reasonable accommodations to individuals with disabilities
MFP	Money Follows the Person	Allows for Medicaid money to be spent on community-based services
ARRA	American Recovery and Reinvestment Act	A stimulus package to increase funding for FMAPs
CFC	Community First Choice	Facilitates LTSS being providing in homes and communities
CLD	Culturally and linguistically diverse	Non-white or minority
ASD	Autism spectrum disorder	A developmental disability impacting communication and social skills
FINDS	Family and Individual Need for Disability Services	A national survey of individuals with disabilities and their families who do not receive formal DD services
MLTSS	Managed long-term services and supports	A managed care organization provides LTSS to individuals with disabilities
DSP	Direct support professionals	Individuals who work directly with people with IDD

Notably, individuals with IDD–including those receiving Medicaid Waiver funded support–are continuing to live in the family home. It is estimated that in 2015, only 683,290 individuals with IDD, roughly 13.5%, lived in a supervised residential setting (i.e., Intermediate Care

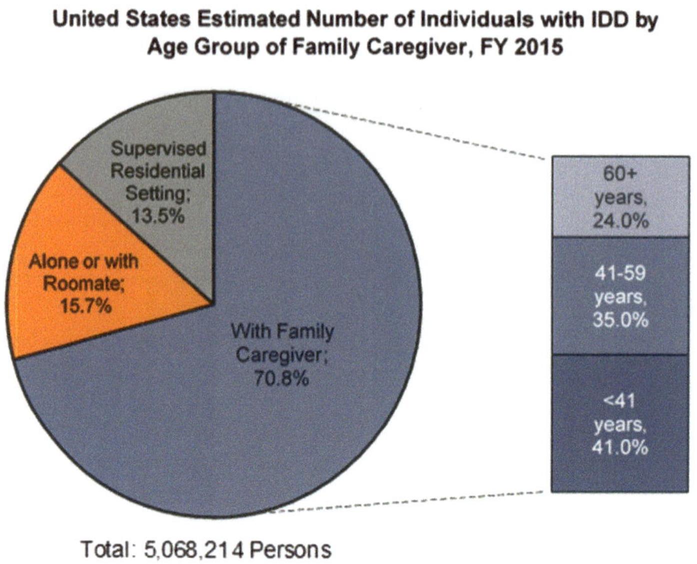

Figure 1 Estimated Number of Individuals with IDD by age group of family caregivers. *Source: Braddock et al. (2017), based on Fujiura, G. T. (2015).*

Facilities for persons with Intellectual Disabilities [ICFs/ID] or Home and Community-Based Services [HCBS] funded settings) while another 793,615 (15.7%) lived on their own or with a roommate. The vast majority of individuals with IDD, an estimated 3.59 million (71%), lived with a family caregiver. Only 17% of these individuals and families received any formal support from state IDD agencies (Braddock et al., 2017). See Fig. 1.

As a result, families continue to be the primary caregivers for individuals with IDD in the United States. Thus, almost 92% of older adults who receive LTSS at home receive family support (i.e., services that support the individual with IDD and the family); further, 66% receive all of their support from their family members (Grossman & Magaña, 2016). Because of the aging population of individuals with IDD and the preference for home and community-based services (versus institutional settings), there is an increased emphasis on family support services (Seltzer & Krauss, 1994). Family support services can help families make informed choices about supports (Turnbull, 2006); family support services are available as part of LTSS.

1. THE EVOLUTION OF COMMUNITY-BASED SUPPORTS

1.1 The Origin of Adult Services and Supports

During America's colonial period, there were no formalized systems of support for people with disabilities as they were mainly cared for by family members. The Protestant Church and Britain's Elizabethan Poor Laws had considerable influence on the attitudes toward the poor, The Church viewed the circumstances of the poor as being due to Providence, or God's will. Widows, the elderly, orphans, individuals with disabilities, and the sick were regarded as being in their respective situations as determined by God and through no fault of their own. Thus, they were considered "deserving poor." The "idle," or those choosing not to work, although seemingly of sound body and mind, were not provided the same type of relief (Rothman, 1990).

At the turn of the 18th century in dense population centers, such as Boston and New York, poor relief became very expensive for local economies. In an effort to lessen the economic impact of relief in urban communities, almshouses were constructed. Over time, however, almshouses began to provide care for individuals without families to rely on or those too sick and "burdensome" to be cared for by a neighbor. Individuals considered to be 'unmanageable,' (e.g., individuals who, in contemporary society, would have acute mental health diagnoses) were housed in the cellars of almshouses or in shacks within city limits (Rothman, 1990). Most of the inhabitants of the early almshouses were individuals with chronic illness or disabilities. By 1800, the urban almshouse was considered "… a home for hopeless causes," (Ferguson, 2004, p. 47), and by the mid-19th century, almshouses became a common treatment for the indigent. Eventually, inhabitants of almshouses were mainly orphans and individuals with disabilities who were considered unable to have contributory roles in the community.

The Industrial Revolution and wartime economy during the early 19th century led to increased internal migration and subsequent urbanization. As a result, many individuals had to seek medical treatment at local hospitals (Engel, 2006). In urban areas, few non-secular or municipal hospitals provided medical treatment for the poor. Barely more than almshouses, they offered little actual medical treatment as few remedies were available (Field, 2007). Hospitals with religious affiliations, initially funded by philanthropy, provided free care to those within their religious, ethnic, cultural, and/or geographic communities, as long as the patient was of the 'deserving poor.' Individuals deemed to be 'undeserving poor,' such as "... the drunkard and the sloth ..." (Engel, 2006, p. 9), were sent to the municipal hospitals for treatment. Municipal hospitals, funded by local and state taxes, were considered mechanisms to maintain public order by removing vagrants and other such 'undesirables' from the city streets (Engel, 2006). Over time, newly constructed municipal hospitals became de facto almshouses.

Hospital stays of individuals without disabilities were temporary, as compared to the elderly and individuals with disabilities who became long-term residents. Extended hospital stays for individuals with disabilities continued until the rise of 'special' schools for 'the feebleminded,' and asylums for the 'insane,', leaving the 'hospitals' to the elderly. By the middle of the 19th century, private schools began to open on the East Coast of the United States, the aim of which was to prepare children with disabilities to live and work in society, thus freeing their families from the burden of their care (Trent, 1994). Schools were situated in isolated rural areas in which it was thought that pupils could escape from societal stressors and unwelcome stares of the public (Wolfensberger, 1975). Other schools opened in Ohio, New York, Illinois, and Pennsylvania (Braddock & Parish, 2002) with the intent to demonstrate that people with intellectual disabilities "... were able to learn and most ... were able to become productive citizens" (Trent, 1994, p. 23).

The Post Civil War depression, however, made it difficult for graduating students to obtain employment as intended; subsequently, many found their way back into almshouses, asylums, or jails. In addition, families affected by the depression could no longer afford private school tuition. The economic downturn made it difficult for families to care for their relatives with disabilities; thus, they were forced to turn them over to the care of the private schools. Because of the decrease in private revenue and the increase in residents, schools struggled to find resources to meet student needs (Trent, 1994). In response, schools changed their focus from training students to supervising 'inmates' (Braddock & Parish, 2002) and allowed the admission of both children and adults with multiple disabilities (Trent, 1994). Schools found themselves with two types of residents: those who had received training but were unable to obtain and/or maintain employment in their communities or whose families would not accept them back into the family household and people who had multiple disabilities for which families were unable to provide care and supervision (Trent, 1994).

In the final quarter of the 19th century, it seemed that such schools had failed (Wolfensberger, 1975). The schools were able to teach the pupils, but not educate them to the level of independence that would allow them to live on their own. Perceiving failure, schools shifted their efforts from education to protection from society (Trent, 1994). Education of the 'feebleminded' came to be seen as a worthless endeavor (Wolfensberger, 1975). Having already been situated in rural areas, some institutions were able to become self-sufficient through farming (Wolfensberger, 1975). Despite this departure from the original intent of the special schools, construction continued. Admission of private pay pupils decreased, while publicly supported charity admissions soared.

It was in this climate that Henry Goddard returned to the United States from Europe in 1908, bringing with him intelligence tests recently developed by Alfred Binet and Theodore Simon. Armed with these tests, Goddard became the first American psychologist to diagnose 'feeblemindedness' (Zenderland, 2004). This tool, many believed, provided scientific validity to the theory of eugenics, or the promotion of the "reproduction of superior human stock" (Trent, 1994, p. 136). Peaking between 1908 and 1915, this ideology positioned individuals with disabilities as social 'menaces' who would eventually turn to crime as a response to the poor morality caused by their 'feeblemindedness' (Wolfensberger, 1975). As such, "... people with disabilities and their families came to be seen as threats to the society ..." (Wilgosh, Sobsey, & Scorgie, 2003, p. 193).

In 1912, Goddard, published *The Kallikak Family: A Study in the Heredity of Feeble-Mindedness,* the story of a young institutionalized woman, pseudonymised Deborah Kallikak (Zenderland, 2004). To many of his contemporaries, Goddard's "... study seemed to suggest a scientific breakthrough in explaining the role played by heredity in causing the mental condition then called 'feeblemindedness'" (Zenderland, 2004, p. 165). Causation, however, continued to baffle Goddard. His thesis of hereditary causation of 'feeblemindedness' was influenced by the works of eugenicist, Francis Galton, geneticist Gregor Mendel, and biologist Charles Davenport (Zenderland, 2004). Goddard traced Deborah's family tree and found that her "... defectiveness was evidenced not only by diminished mental capacity but also by social incapacity, for Deborah's relatives included numerous paupers, prostitutes, and petty criminals" (Zenderland, 2004, p. 175). Goddard used this 'evidence' regarding 'feeblemindedness' as a genetic trait, manageable through prevention or procreation, to justify segregation and sterilization.

Such beliefs became popular justifications for institutionalization intending to prohibit the procreation of individuals with disabilities through segregation of the sexes and sterilization. Society believed it could rid itself of 'defectives', which would, in turn, reduce public expenditures for their care over time (Wolfensberger, 1975). 'Feeblemindedness' came to be viewed as a social burden, which could be relieved through tax-financed institutional care fueling an increase in the construction and utilization of institutions. By 1923, there were 138 public and private facilities for people with I/DD (Trent, 1994). Similar to the post-Civil War Era, more families chose to institutionalize their relatives with I/DD during the Great Depression as unemployment and poverty made it difficult for families to provide care (Braddock & Parish, 2002). Such continued perceptions of individuals with IDD as abnormal and deviant strongly influenced not only societal attitudes but also treatment (Lakin, Bruininks, & Sigford, 1981).

Family Influence. As World War II came to an end, it became apparent that the Nazi euthanasia program was borne of American eugenic ideology. The "crimes against humanity" (Wilgosh et al., 2003, p. 197) committed during the Holocaust, which included individuals with disabilities, fueled discussion among parents of children with disabilities who spoke out about the 'worthiness' of the lives of their offspring with disabilities (Wilgosh et al., 2003). Nobel Prize winning author, Pearl Buck, penned three books that framed children with disabilities in a positive light. In her 1965 book, *The Gifts They Bring*, she presented the "positive contributions that these children brought to their families" (Wilgosh, et al., 2003, p. 198). Dale Evans Rogers, wife of the singer/actor Roy Rogers, wrote *Angel Unaware* in 1953 encapsulating the Rogers' family experience of the loss of Robin, their daughter with Down syndrome. The book advocated for families to raise their offspring with disabilities in their homes and "dared to suggest that they actually can be good for families" (Wilgosh et al., 2003, p. 198). Such 'confessional literature' (Trent, 1994) "allowed … parents to discuss their disabled children as valuable and contributing members of their families …" (Brockley, 2004, p. 151).

It was within this new paradigm, coupled with the post-World War II baby boom and improvements in medical technology–which increased the survival rate of children born with congenital disabilities–that individuals with IDD gained recognition within the general population (Farber, 1968). In addition, IDD was affecting more middle and upper class families, weakening the prior belief that IDD was only a problem among families of lower socio-economic status and, thus, propelling individuals with IDD to gain higher recognition as a social concern.

As early as 1933, parents of children with IDD formed an association in Ohio called the Council for Retarded Children (sic). Similar groups formed across the United States comprised of parents whose children had not been included in the public school systems. The local groups came together in 1950 to form a federation called the National Association of Parents and Friends of Mentally Retarded Children (sic) (later called the National Association for Retarded Children, or NARC). By 1965, the number of local affiliates numbered over one thousand. The primary objective of parent groups such as NARC, presently called The Arc, was to create special schools for their children with significant IDD. Later, The Arc expanded to include other services (Farber, 1968).

The Arc created safe spaces for families to include their children with IDD, regardless of whether they lived in an institution or the family home, in activities approximating the typical middle class family such as holiday parties, summer camp and swim class. Schooling, however, was still unavailable to all but 'educably mentally retarded' (*sic*). Parent groups attempted to fill the gap in the availability of education to their children with significant ID by forming private, special schools (Jones, 2004), which operated out of church basements and vacant schools (Metzel, 2004). As parents became more politically active, many advocated for special classrooms within their local public schools (Jones, 2004).

The post-WWII parent movement quickly and significantly altered the perceptions of individuals with IDD and how those perceptions were relayed in the media and other public venues (Castles, 2004). In this context, President Kennedy issued a statement regarding the need for a national plan for individuals with ID. To facilitate this plan, he called together a group of "outstanding physicians, scientists, educators, lawyers, psychologists, social scientists, and leaders in the field," (The President's Panel on Mental Retardation, October 1962, p. 201) to form the President's Panel on Mental Retardation (now the President's Committee for People with Intellectual Disabilities). The Panel was tasked with exploring prevention and cure, studying relevant factors, evaluating available programs, identifying gaps and failures, as well as formulating recommendations with regard to major areas of concern, present programs, needed personnel, and governmental/private efforts to ameliorate IDD. President Kennedy was not acting only as Commander in Chief, but as a brother. His sister, Rosemary Kennedy, had a significant ID (Trent, 1994). As a result of such national attention, ID was becoming less feared; however, it was still widely believed that it was in the best interest for the health and well-being of the family for the individual with IDD to be removed from the home (Brockley, 2004).

In December of 1965, Blatt and Kaplan visited five institutions for individuals with IDD (Blatt & Kaplan, 1974). During their tours of the facilities, Kaplan, a free-lance photographer, secretly snapped photos of what they observed and published them in the late summer of 1966 as a photographic essay entitled *Christmas in Purgatory*. As a result, the 1970 *Wyatt v. Stickney* lawsuit exposed deplorable living conditions at Bryce State Hospital in Tuscaloosa, Alabama. Two years later, in 1972, Geraldo Rivera's exposé at Willowbrook State School on Staten Island in New York revealed to the nation on a major television network the horrible living conditions of individuals with disabilities (Rothman & Rothman, 2005).

Policy influence. Prior to the creation of Medicaid in 1965, states used local funds to finance disability services (Prouty, Smith, & Lakin, 2007; U.S. Department of Health and Human Services, 2000). After years of legislative efforts (e.g., the 1957 Forand Bill and the Kerr-Mills bill in 1960), the Medicaid program was created through amending the Social Security Act establishing a state-federal government entitlement program, which provides a legal right to services to those who meet eligibility criteria. In 1971, a provision was added in which Medicaid reimburses state spending for services rendered through reimbursement formulas using each state's Federal Medical Assistance Percentage (FMAP), based on state per capita personal income (Braddock et al., 2005).

Today, there are three major areas covered under the Medicaid program: provision of health insurance for low-income Americans, long-term care for older Americans, and specialized services and long-term care for individuals with disabilities (Hemp & Braddock, 2003). States are afforded flexibility within the Medicaid program to determine the type, amount, duration, and scope of services provided (Centers for Medicare and Medicaid Services, 2007). There are, however, certain services that are mandated by federal Medicaid law. Table 2, reproduced from Lulinski Norris (2008), displays summaries of the mandatory and optional categories in Medicaid. Of note, the Medicaid program does provide funding for long-term care. However, it is only mandated for provision in skilled nursing facilities. The two core Medicaid programs for individuals with IDD are ICF/IDs and the HCBS Waiver, both of which fall into the optional services category.

Table 2 Mandatory and Optional Medicaid Services

	Health Care
Mandatory Services	**Optional Services**
Certified pediatric and family nurse practitioner services	Medical or remedial care provided by state licensed practitioners
Laboratory and x-ray services	Prescription drugs
Early and Periodic Screening, Diagnosis, and Treatment (EPSDT) for individuals <21	Diagnostic, screening, preventative, and rehabilitative services
In/outpatient hospital services	Primary care case management services
Family planning services and supplies	Dental services
Health center services	Physical therapy and related services
Rural health clinic services	Prosthetics and eyeglasses
Nurse midwife services	TB related services
Vaccinations for children	Transportation services
Physician services	Targeted case management services
	Long Term Care
Mandatory Services	**Optional Services**
Skilled Nursing facility (SNF) services for people >21	Inpatient hospital and NF services for individuals 65+ in an Institute for Mental Disease (IMD)
Home health care services for those entitled to nursing facility services	ICF/ID services
	Inpatient psychiatric hospital services for individuals 21+
	Home health care
	Case management
	Respiratory Care services for ventilator-dependent
	Personal care services
	Private duty nursing
	Hospice
	Services under Program of All-Inclusive Care for the Elderly (PACE)
	HCBS Waiver

Sources: Braddock, Hemp, & Rizzolo (2003) and Centers for Medicare and Medicaid Services (2007).

Media attention from the Wyatt v. Stickney case and the Willowbrook exposé led to the adoption of regulatory standards. The ICF/ID program was added in 1971 by Section 1905(d) of the Social Security Act. An ICF/ID program is an optional residential benefit provided in a state-licensed and certified facility to individuals with ID who require active treatment (Centers for Medicare and Medicaid Services, 2018a, 2018b). Reimbursement for services provided is contingent on eight conditions of participation: (1) facility regulations with regard to governing body and management; (2) client protections; (3) facility staffing; (4) active treatment; (5) client behavior and facility practices; (6) health care services; (7) physical environment; and (8) dietetic services (Requirements for States and Long Term Care Facilities, 1988).

In FY 2015, there were 78,138 people living in ICFs/ID representing 11.5% of all people with IDD living outside of the family home at a total cost of $11 billion (Braddock et al., 2017). In terms of annual per person costs, publicly-operated ICFs/ID for 16 or more people averaged $210,110 per year, while privately-operated ICFs/ID for 16 or more was $113,744. Publicly-operated ICFs/ID for less than 16 people averaged $165,054 per person per year while privately-operated ICFs/ID averaged $106,553 (Braddock et al., 2017).

In 1981, the HCBS Waiver program was created to address both the rising cost of skilled nursing care and the institutional bias of Medicaid, which meant that to receive any residential services, a person had to reside in one of two congregate settings: a skilled nursing facility or an ICF/ID. HCBS created an alternative to institutional care by waiving three main provisions in the Social Security Act and, thus, allowing services to be provided in community settings: (1) 'statewideness,' which requires the program to be offered statewide allowing states to target particular areas; (2) comparability of services, which requires availability of services for all Medicaid eligible persons thus allowing states to make waiver services available to those at risk of being institutionalized; and (3) income and resource rules allowing states to provide Medicaid services to those who would otherwise be eligible for an institutional setting (Centers for Medicare and Medicaid Services, 2008). Waiver services must be cost-neutral meaning that they cannot cost more, on average, than institutional services. Services covered under the HCBS Waiver include: case management (i.e., service coordination), personal assistance (i.e., homemaker, home health aide, and personal care attendant), adult day health services, habilitation (both day and residential), and respite care. Additionally, states can propose other types of services that may assist in maintaining individuals in their community homes rather than diverting them to institutional settings (Centers for Medicare and Medicaid Services, 2014a, 2014b, 2014c). For inclusion in the HCBS waiver program, the state must assure the following: (1) waiver services cost less, on average, than institutional care; (2) protection of the health and welfare of individuals served; (3) standards meet the needs of the population served; and (4) services are provided in accordance with a plan of care (Centers for Medicare and Medicaid Services, 2008). States have choice over the number and types of waiver programs as well as the number of individuals with IDD who are enrolled. In 2018, there were 531 waiver programs available for persons with HIV/AIDS, traumatic brain injury, cystic fibrosis, mental illness, Alzheimer's disease, physical disabilities, persons that are technologically dependent, as well as persons with IDD (Centers for Medicare and Medicaid Services, 2018a, 2018b). As such, state Medicaid programs vary greatly from state to state.

1.2 Deinstitutionalization Outcomes

For decades, researchers have explored changes in individual behaviors as a result of deinstitutionalization and have overwhelming evidence that individuals moving from institutions to community-based settings display an increase in adaptive behavior as compared to their institutionalized counterparts (Larson & Lakin, 1989) and that people benefit from moving to the community from an institution (Kim, Larson, & Lakin, 1999).

Early studies reported that differences in environments produce different outcomes for individuals moving out of institutions (Bjaanes & Butler, 1974). For example, environments that were more "normalized" (versus institutional) were more likely to increase the independent living skills of the residents with IDD (Seltzer, 1981). Quality of life was better on average and care was "more adequate" (p. 122) in smaller community-based settings (Balla, 1976). Further, in community-based (versus institutional) settings, individuals experience better outcomes related to adaptive behavior, increased self-determination, community participation and friendships with peers without disabilities (Heller, 2002). In fact, smaller (versus larger) settings offer more community involvement, larger social networks, more friends, greater opportunities for choice and self-determination, a higher quality of life, and increased satisfaction of residents and their families (Kozma, Mansell, & Beadle-Brown, 2009).

The provision of the HCBS Waiver allows states to provide individuals with disabilities the option of receiving community-integrated services rather than segregated institutional care. The number of Waiver programs available as well as the scope of and spending on such programs indicate a trend toward provision of services in the community. In fact, since the early 1980's, amendments to federal laws and policies have been chipping away at Medicaid's institutional bias and making way for funding options for home and community-based long-term care alternatives. The HCBS Waiver "... has been an essential part of community services expansion in the states ..." (Braddock et al., 2005, p. 28). Incorporation of the federal match under the Medicaid program has allowed states to offer an array of Medicaid funded community-based services to individuals with IDD who would otherwise require institutional admission to skilled nursing, intermediate, or ICF/ID facilities.

1.3 System Rebalancing

Since peaking at 194,650 in 1967 (Department of Health, Education, and Welfare, 1972), the census of publicly-operated IDD institutions has dropped to 21,103 (89.2% decrease) in FY 2015 at an average annual rate of 4%, resulting in the closure or in process closure of 173 public institutions (Braddock et al., 2017). Much of the rebalancing completed in the United States has been the result of advocacy, class action litigation, including *Olmstead* cases, waiting list cases, and access to Medicaid benefits cases (Braddock et al., 2013).

Litigation. The *Olmstead* Decision of 1999 was issued by the United States Supreme Court (*Olmstead v. L.C.,* 1999) in response to a lawsuit brought by Lois Curtis and Elaine Wilson in 1995 (Bazelon Center for Mental Health Law, 2009). Both women had a dual diagnosis (i.e., developmental disability and mental illness) and were voluntarily admitted to Georgia Regional Hospital's psychiatric unit (*Olmstead*, 1999). After receiving clearance from professionals, neither woman was granted their desired community placement (Bazelon, 2009). The court rejected the state's claim of inadequate funding for community placement and ruled this was a violation of Title II of the Americans with Disabilities Act (ADA) of 1990 (*Olmstead*, 1999). Title II states, "A public entity shall administer services, programs, and activities in the most integrated setting appropriate to the needs of qualified individuals with disabilities" [28 CFR § 35.130(d)]. *Olmstead* found states are to comply with Title II of the ADA to avoid discriminatory practices of institutionalization when community-based alternatives would be appropriate (Ng, Wong, & Harrington, 2012). As of May of 2013, Ng, Wong, and Harrington (2013) reported a total of 193 *Olmstead*-related cases in all but five states (i.e., Iowa, Idaho, North Dakota, South Dakota, and Vermont) and the District of Columbia.

Policy. Money Follows the Person (MFP) was initially authorized by the Deficit Reduction Act of 2005 with the purpose of providing states with assistance to balance LTSS spending with HCBS waiver spending by assisting Medicaid recipients to transition to communities from institutions (Centers for Medicare and Medicaid Services, 2014a, 2014b, 2014c). MFP acknowledges the institutional bias of Medicaid and allows for money that was intended to be spent on institutional services to 'follow' the person into a community-based option and allows for assistance with the costs associated with that transition. Federal MFP funds were not to exceed $1.75 billion through FY 2011. However, funds were extended through September 30, 2016 by the Patient Protection and Affordable Care Act of 2010. The extension included $2.25 billion from FY 2012 through 2016. As of December 2013, 7487 individuals with IDD transitioned to a community placement from an institutional setting at a cost savings of $361 million. Without the provision of MFP, 50% of MFP participants with IDD would not have transitioned into the community (Irvin et al., 2017). MFP funding allocation expired on September 30, 2016. However, legislation has been introduced to continue the program. Specifically, Senate Bill 2227, the bipartisan "Ensuring Medicaid Provides Opportunities for Widespread Equity, Resources, and Care Act" (EMPOWER Care Act) was introduced by Senators Portman (R-OH) and Cantwell (D-WA) on December 13, 2017. A bipartisan companion bill was introduced in the House on March 15, 2018 as H.R. 5306 by Representatives Gruthrie (KY 2nd – R) and Dingell (MI 12th - D).

The American Recovery and Reinvestment Act of 2009 (ARRA), signed into law in February of 2009, provided an economic stimulus including a temporary increase in state FMAPs to provide relief from increased medical expenditures during the recessionary period (Association of University Centers on Disabilities, 2010a). The FMAP increase was retroactively effective October 1, 2008 and intended to last for nine quarters, ending December 31, 2010. In August of 2010, due to the continued economic recession, however, the FMAP increase was extended an additional six months through June of 2011. The increased FMAP extension was critical to Medicaid service provision, particularly during the Great Recession, as Medicaid utilization has an inverse relation with the economy. The Great Recession, which occurred in 2007—09, saw an increase in unemployment and an increase in Medicaid beneficiaries coupled with a decrease in state revenues (Holahan & Chen, 2011) that created a gap between revenues and spending (Kaiser Commission on Medicaid and the Uninsured, 2011).

The Patient Protection and Affordable Care Act of 2010, which was signed into law on March 23, 2010 by President Obama and implemented in October of 2011, created the optional Community First Choice (CFC) benefit through amendment of the Social Security Act via the addition of section 1915(k). CFC is intended to contribute to the rebalancing of LTSS spending by providing LTSS in individual homes and communities as opposed to institutional settings (Department of Health and Human Services, 2015). All eligible persons (i.e., individuals that would otherwise require an institutional level of care and meet income requirements) must receive benefits under this option should they require them. States are not mandated to provide this option; however, a 6% increase was added to the FMAP of states that have an approved plan. In 2018, five states were approved to offer this option (Centers for Medicare and Medicaid Services, 2018a, 2018b).

Large congregate settings were the predominant place of residence for a majority of individuals with IDD who lived outside of the family home up until the later part of the 19th century; censuses of such facilities peaked in 1967 at 194,650 (Braddock et al., 2017; US Department of Health, Education, and Welfare, 1972). Over 20 years later in 1989, the number of individuals with IDD living in community-based settings for six or fewer people surpassed the number of people with IDD living in institutional settings (Braddock et al., 2015). This shift would not have been possible without the creation of and subsequent amendments to the Social Security Act. In FY 2015, there were 115 waiver programs in 46 states and the District of Columbia that provided 741,285 people with IDD supports totaling $34.5 billion at an average cost of $46,481 per person annually (Braddock et al., 2017; Friedman, 2017).

2. FAMILY SYSTEMS THEORY

Over the last half century, shifts in research, policy, and practice have helped create opportunities in education, employment, community living, and a quality of life. While there has been significant progress in transforming systems that support individuals with IDD to have equal access to a meaningful life in the community, the role and needs of the family in achieving this have not been fully recognized or supported in disability policy or practice (Reynolds, Gotto, Agosta, Arnold, & Fay, 2016).

Since the 1980s, there has been a growing recognition of the critical role of the family in the system of long term care for individuals with IDD. This recognition has resulted in service delivery that is progressively more family-centered (e.g., Part C or early intervention of the Individuals with Disabilities Education Act). Placing the individual within the context of their family system, family-centered service delivery is characterized by family choice, family strengths, and the family as the unit of support (Turnbull, Turbiville, & Turnbull, 2000).

Derived from General Systems Theory (Von Bertalanffy, 1969), family systems theory is predicated on the assumption that individuals cannot be fully understood in isolation or outside their family context (e.g., Whitchurch & Constantine, 1993). As such, the theory suggests that families, like mechanical systems, act as interconnected and holistic systems of individuals. Because of the interdependence of such relationships, individual dynamics or changes directly affect systems in their entirety (Whitchurch & Constantine, 1993) – this interdependence is complex. When one member does not function well, all other members in the system are impacted. Further, the family interacts with other systems, including those that provide additional services or benefits to the individual (e.g., social security administration, health care).

Family Systems Theory and Adult Services. Due to the interconnectedness and interdependence of individuals within family systems, it is erroneous to conceptualize LTSS as affecting only the individual with IDD. These relationships are interrelated in a circular, recursive manner such that the actions and influences of one member of a system cannot help but affect other members as well. In this way, while the services and benefits may be provided to one family member, it is inevitable that the other family members and relationships within the system as a whole will be affected. Relational functions between family members will affect how the individual copes, responds, manages, and makes meaning of the supports and services received. Consequently, to gain a more comprehensive understanding of the outcomes of LTSS, it is imperative to view such experiences through the lens of family systems theory.

Family systems theory eschews the traditional, reductionist, individual model of supports and services to focus on the interactional approach, which recognizes the combined influence of multiple factors on any given phenomenon (Steinglass, 1987). When applying this perspective to LTSS, it becomes evident that it is not solely individual outcomes that should be assessed. Contextual and environmental factors in the individual's life, family background, belief systems subscribed to, and aspects of current relationships (among other things) also impact long-term outcomes. In the same way, the functioning of family relationships is determined by the residential presence or absence of an individual with IDD as well as other factors, creating an interactional effect that impacts long term outcomes.

To this end, family systems theory posits that systems adjust and reorganize themselves to maintain homeostasis to ensure continuity of functioning (Becvar & Becvar, 1999; Steinglass, 1987). Positive feedback occurs within systems when a change has occurred, signaling members that action must be taken to re-establish the status quo (Becvar & Becvar, 1999). Members typically respond to positive feedback by altering their own behaviors in an effort to alter the behaviors of others and restore balance in the relationship. Thus, within the context of adult services, when LTSS are provided to an individual with IDD, the entire family is impacted and must react by changing their own behaviors to facilitate the behaviors of the individual with IDD. For example, if an individual with IDD receives LTSS, the family must identify, obtain, coordinate, and monitor such services.

3. CAREGIVING CONTEXTS AMONG FAMILIES OF INDIVIDUALS WITH IDD

In light of family systems theory and LTSS as well as the longer lives of individuals with IDD, it is crucial to explore the caregiving contexts among families of individuals with IDD. Parents of individuals with IDD face the unique circumstance of "lifespan parenting" —active caregiving from birth until either the parent's death or the death of the child. Even when individuals with IDD do not reside in the family home, caregiving is considered a lifelong experience. Although many parents report positive outcomes associated with their caregiving roles, research also indicates there are negative impacts on the well-being of these families (Brown et al., 2003; Greenberg, Seltzer, & Greenley, 1993; Jokinen & Brown, 2011). Lifelong caregiving leads to various stressors for parents as well as siblings, who are often enlisted to care for family members when parents are no longer able (Burke, Taylor, Urbano, & Hodapp, 2012; Jokinen & Brown, 2011; Werner, Edwards, & Baum, 2009). Specifically, it is important to consider lifespan parenting among different contexts including aging caregivers, sibling caregivers, culture, co-residence, and families without formal adult services.

3.1 Aging Caregivers of Individuals With IDD

With over 70% of individuals with IDD living in the family home and 24% of these caregivers aged 60 or over (Braddock et al., 2017), the issue of aging caregivers warrants our attention as many of the needs of both the aging caregiver and the individual with IDD change across the life course. Perkins and van Heumen (2016) draw on their own research and that of colleagues to highlight the physical, psychological, and social issues unique to aging caregivers of individuals with IDD. Physical issues include the emergence of age-related health issues in both caregivers and individuals with IDD. The physical demands of providing direct care (e.g., bathing, dressing) become more difficult with age. Likewise, new health conditions, such as heart disease and diabetes, demand significant care requirements on top of already existing needs. Using population data, Seltzer, Floyd, Song, Greenberg, and Hong (2011) examined patterns of attainment, social participation, psychological functioning, and health in parents of adults with and without IDD during their early 50s and mid 60s. Few differences between parent groups were seen in regards to psychological well-being, and health. However, poorer physical health and worse mental health outcomes emerged at early old age (i.e., mid 60s) among parents of children with (versus without) IDD with even more distinct differences noted when examining the residential status of the adult with IDD (i.e., co-residence with parents compared to adults with IDD living elsewhere). Specifically, when co-residing, health outcomes were worse. Thus, similar to the greater likelihood of off-time or missed milestones (e.g., obtaining a driver's license, moving out of the family home) experienced by their children with IDD (Jones, 2012), the life course trajectory of parents of adults with IDD and normative transitions of aging differ from their peers who are not tasked with caregiving. Many parents of adults with (versus without) IDD may never experience the "empty nest" (Seltzer & Krauss, 1994) and often remain engaged in daily parenting and caregiving responsibilities leaving little time to develop new interests or engage socially with others (Seltzer et al., 2011). Even with increasing physical demands and the emergence of significant health conditions for both caregivers and individuals with IDD, many caregivers who have provided decades of support to their family member struggle to ask for help. As individuals with IDD are remaining in the family home (Braddock et al., 2017) and having longer lives (see Bittles et al., 2002), planning for a time when someone else may need to become the primary caregiver of the individual with IDD is a difficult and relatively new psychological issue that families must address.

3.2 Sibling Caregivers of Individuals With IDD

Siblings often have the longest familial relationships with one another (Cicirelli, 2000). As parents age and are less able to caregive for their family members with IDD, siblings are often looked to as the next generation of caregivers (Heller & Arnold, 2010). Indeed, many siblings of individuals with IDD report anticipating fulfilling caregiving roles (Burke et al., 2012). Although studies range with respect to the percentage of sibling caregivers, most studies expect 20–51% of siblings to fulfill caregiving roles (Lee & Burke, 2018). Notably, most sibling studies reflect convenience samples of White, female, highly involved siblings (Hodapp, Glidden, & Kaiser, 2005; Lee & Burke, 2018). Thus, the actual population percentage of sibling caregivers may vary.

Consistent in the research, however, is the concern siblings have about their impending caregiving roles in relation to the availability of adult services and future planning. Regarding the former, many studies report that siblings are concerned about navigating the adult service delivery system on behalf of their brothers and sisters with IDD (Arnold, Heller, & Kramer, 2012; Burke, Fish, & Lawton, 2015). Unlike their parents, siblings are starting from scratch to understand how to access services. Although they may not have the same knowledge as their parents about adult services, siblings have witnessed their parents express frustration with accessing services (Burke et al., 2015). As a result, siblings are worried about learning to navigate service delivery systems when they transition to caregiving roles. For example, in a study with 139 siblings of adults with DD, Arnold et al. (2012) asked sibling respondents about their support needs. Three themes emerged: needing disability-related information; receiving support for their caregiving roles; and enhancing the formal support system. Indeed, each of these support needs relate to services and supports for individuals with IDD and their families. Further, the concern about adult services is warranted as when siblings are unable to access services, they are less able to protect the rights of their brothers and sisters with IDD (Heller & Factor, 1994).

Hand-in-hand with the apprehension of navigating service delivery systems and future caregiving roles, siblings are also concerned about future planning (i.e., conducting a set of activities to ensure supports are available for individuals with IDD in the future). Siblings report wanting to conduct future planning to ensure seamless transitions to caregiving roles (Heller & Arnold, 2010; Heller & Kramer, 2009). In addition, parents also report wanting to participate in future planning (Bowey & McGlaughlin, 2007). However, less than half of families of adults with IDD report engaging in future planning (Anderson et al., 2018; Davys, Mitchell, & Haigh, 2010; Freedman, Krauss, & Seltzer, 1997; Heller & Factor, 1993). Notably, future planning includes adult services as siblings must consider the residential living and employment of their brothers and sisters with IDD. To date, no empirically-based interventions about future planning have focused exclusively on the needs of adult siblings of individuals with IDD (Lee, 2018, in preparation). Siblings are apt to be concerned about future planning as without future planning, individuals with IDD are vulnerable to crisis situations and institutional settings (Hewitt et al., 2013a; Thompson & Wright, 2001). For family members—including parents and siblings—the lack of future planning can induce anxiety (Smith, Tobin, & Fullmer, 1995).

3.3 Cultural Contexts

In the research about families of adults with IDD, most research focuses on White families (Harry, 2002). Of the limited extant research, studies often combine minority families into the category *culturally and linguistically diverse* (i.e., CLD, non-White families, Harry, 2002; Burke & Heller, 2017). Thus, individual cultural differences are largely ignored. However, culture clearly impacts individuals with IDD, their families, and their access to services. Regarding the latter, minority (versus White) families are significantly less likely to receive needed adult services (Burke & Heller, 2017; Balcazar, Oberoi, Suarez-Balcazar, & Alvarado, 2012).

Although we could review the impact of culture across many different families, for the sake of brevity, we will highlight the cultural context of African American and Latino families of adults with IDD. Before delving into specific cultural contexts, it is important to mention intersectionality. Indeed, CLD families may have multiple minoritizing identities in relation to race, class, and disability (Erevelles & Minnear, 2010). A single characteristic (e.g., race or ethnicity) cannot explain all experiences; intersectionality can help explain how multiple characteristics interact with one another (Pastrana, 2004). Thus, in the context of CLD families of individuals with IDD, intersectionality is crucial as individuals with IDD are more likely to reflect minority (Harry, 2002) and low-income backgrounds (Emerson, 2007). Within this section, the reader should keep in mind these multiple factors.

African American Families of Adults with IDD. Compared to White families, African American families of adults with IDD are more likely to face unmet service needs and, correspondingly, receive less services (Pruchno & McMullen, 2004; Bershadsky et al., 2014). Perhaps in response to unmet service needs, African American families are more likely to rely on family members and social networks than formal supports (Grossman & Magaña, 2016). This reliance on natural (versus paid or formal) supports may stem from negative experiences with previous service delivery systems (e.g., the school system, Williams, 2007) and mistrust of professionals (Hess, Molina, & Kozleski, 2006). Also, family members and friends who reflect the same ethnic or racial background may be more understanding of the experience of being a minority (in this case, African American) in the United States (Hanline & Daley, 1992).

Further, African Americans are often very connected to spirituality (Scharlach, Giunta, Chow, & Lehning, 2008). Indeed, religion is recognized as a basic value of African American families (Scharlach et al., 2008). Among African American families of offspring with IDD, religion and church support (i.e., natural supports) have a significant and positive relation with family adjustment. Unlike traditional service delivery systems, which rely on formal eligibility schemes, religion offers an inclusive mentality of disability (Boyd & Correa, 2005). Because of the restrictive, label-based framing of disability by adult service delivery systems, such systems may be culturally unresponsive. Indeed, adult service delivery systems may be more effective in supporting individuals with IDD and their families when they consider both formal and natural supports as critical to the well-being of the family system.

Latino Families of Adults with IDD. Compared to White families, Latino families of adults with IDD are also more likely to struggle to access services (Mercadente, Evans-Lacko, & Paula, 2009). Further, Latino (versus White) families are more likely to engage in lifespan parenting as they are more likely to have their offspring with IDD stay within the family home for longer periods of time (Blacher, 2001). Indeed, cultural values may facilitate lifespan parenting in Latino families. For example, familism is a common characteristic among Latino families wherein family members have strong loyalty and reciprocity to one another (Magaña & Smith, 2008). Specifically, especially within the disability context, familism includes providing ongoing support to a family member. Because of familism, Latino families may be less interested in their offspring with IDD living outside of the home and more interested in receiving services within the family home. Compared to White families of young adults with ASD, Latino families of young adults with ASD are more satisfied with their family member living in the family home (Magaña and Smith, 2006a, 2006b).

It is also important to recognize that Latino (versus White) families of adults with IDD may experience worse health and, correspondingly, also need services and supports. Although most adult services are aimed at the individual with IDD, especially given the interdependent nature of Latino families, it may also be appropriate to think about supports for their families. For example, Latina mothers may be more likely to focus on the needs of their offspring than their own needs (Rueda, Monzo, Shapiro, Gomez, & Blacher, 2005). As a result, Latino (versus White) families are often in worse physical health and have higher levels of depressions (Magaña and Smith, 2006a, 2006b; 2008; Blacher, Lopez, Shapiro, & Fusco, 1997).

Co-Residence. Many caregiving families co-reside with their adult family member with IDD. In FY 2015, 71% of individuals with IDD lived with their family caregivers (Braddock et al., 2017). Further, many families of adults with IDD choose to live with their family member with IDD even when residential placements are available (Heller, Miller, & Factor, 1997). However, there are challenges with co-residence. For example, when parents co-reside (versus do not co-reside) with their adult family members with ASD, parents rate their situations more negatively (Krauss, Seltzer, & Jacobson, 2005). Further, co-residence is significantly associated with lower marital stability, reduced leisure time, and greater limitations in parent activities of daily life (Seltzer et al., 2011).

Families Without Formal Adult Services. Over the past decade, efforts have been made to capture data about individuals and families who are not receiving any formal DD services through the Family and Individual Need for Disability Services (FINDS) Survey (Anderson et al., 2018). Data collected in 2017 provide a snapshot of these families, although the data are not representative of the general population. Survey results indicated that families, on average, provide over 57 h of care per week to both children and adults with IDD (ranging from nine or fewer to over 80 h per week). Fifty-two percent of respondents reported providing more than 40 h of care per week to their adult family members with IDD. Only 15% reported receiving pay for the provision of support. Half of the caregivers (50%) reported providing support with three or more activities of daily living (e.g., dressing, eating, toileting, grooming, and mobility).

In addition to providing these supports, almost ⅔ of the caregivers reported working; over half (55%) reported working in excess of 40 h per week. The majority (95%) reported that caregiving had an impact on their work such as taking time off, cutting back on work hours, taking a leave of absence, and leaving the workforce. Those who remained employed reported turning down a promotion, passing on career opportunities in another state due to lack of Medicaid portability, and receiving warnings about work attendance or performance. Overwhelmingly, caregivers reported difficulty finding direct support professionals (92%) and respite supports (92%). Unsurprisingly, 85% of caregivers indicated they had challenges in balancing work and caregiving responsibilities.

3.4 Family Caregiving Outcomes

Unsurprisingly, there are benefits and challenges for families of adults with IDD. Benefits include, for example, increased mastery and expertise, and feelings of finding contentment and purpose in life (Haley & Perkins, 2004). However, there are also potential negative outcomes. Indeed, such benefits may help offset some of the "wear and tear" of caregiving. Drawing on the gerontology literature, the wear and tear hypothesis posits that exposure to ongoing life challenges may lead to increased vulnerability and worse health (Pearlin, Menaghen, Lieberman, & Mullan, 1981). Below, we summarize caregiving outcomes with respect to physical health, emotional well-being, and finances.

3.5 Physical Health

The literature about the impact of family caregiving for an adult with IDD on physical health is mixed. A systematic review of 24 studies about family caregiver outcomes found mixed results with respect to physical health (Williamson & Perkins, 2014). Some studies found that, compared to non-caregivers, caregivers of adults with IDD report worse physical health (Burke & Fujiura, 2013) whereas other studies reported that caregivers had better health (Chen, Ryan-Henry, Heller, & Chen, 2001). Further still, some studies found no difference in physical health (Schulz, O'Brien, Bookwala, & Fleissner, 1995). Some of the mixed findings are reflected within individual studies. For example, Yamaki et al. (2009) found that mothers of individuals with (versus without) IDD reported better overall health; however, mothers of individuals with (versus without) IDD also reported a significantly greater number of health conditions. The repercussions of worse caregiver health may impact their family members with IDD. When family caregivers are in worse health, they may provide poor caregiving (Navaie-Waliser et al., 2002).

3.6 Psychological Well-Being

Many studies have found worse psychological well-being among family caregivers of adults with IDD in comparison to non-caregivers (e.g., Anderson et al., 2018; Seltzer et al., 2011; Bourke-Taylor, Pallant, Law, & Howie, 2012; Pinquart & Sörensen, 2007). Specifically, caregiving can lead to increases in: depression, stress, and psychiatric problems (Davis & Carter, 2008). For example, in a national study of 3169 caregivers, nine out of ten caregivers reported being stressed (Anderson et al., 2018). In addition, families may lack the social support to improve their well-being as caregivers have less leisure and social time (Gilleard, Gilleard, Gledhill, & Whittick, 1984) and less social participation (Mailick Seltzer, Greenberg, Floyd, Pettee, & Hong, 2001).

3.7 Finances Well-Being

The literature seems to be consistent in that there is a negative impact on the financial well-being of family caregivers of adults with IDD (for a review, see Williamson & Perkins, 2014). In a national study of 3169 caregivers, 92% of the respondents reported paying out-of-pocket expenses related to their relative's disability (Anderson et al., 2018). Specifically, 67% reported paying more $1000 per year in out-of-pocket expenses while 36% reported expenses greater than $5000 per year. Indeed, caregivers themselves acknowledge the negative impact on their financial state (Seltzer et al., 2011). For example, for an individual with ID, an annual measure of out-of-pocket expenses was $6348 for a household with a pre-tax income of $37,657. Notably, however, among caregivers receiving supports and services (versus caregivers who do not receive supports and services), there is a significant reduction in family out-of-pocket expenses (Caldwell, 2006).

3.8 Compound Caregiving

It is important to note the increased prevalence of compound caregivers—individuals who take care of their family member with IDD as well as another family member (Perkins, 2010). In a study of 91 caregivers of adults with IDD, 37% were current compound caregivers (Perkins & Haley, 2010).

Notably, 66% had been or were currently compound caregivers. Further, caregivers spent 39 h per week on caregiving tasks; compound caregivers spent an additional 12 h a week in their caregiving roles. Thus, it is not surprising that compound caregivers struggled to have personal time and adequate help from others.

4. DISCUSSION

4.1 Contemporary Issues

Below, we highlight contemporary issues, including policy, research, and practice implications, which stem from the above text. Specifically, we discuss: inclusion as a fundamental human right, the transdisciplinary nature of aging and disability, family advocacy, the ongoing co-residence of adults with IDD and their families, and individuals with IDD and their families who do not receive formal services.

4.2 Inclusion Is a Fundamental Human Right

Implications for Research and Practice. Although the history of individuals with IDD has been cemented in institutional and non-inclusive settings, recently, individuals 1with IDD have been living inclusively, within the community. Indeed, recent litigation (i.e., the *Olmstead* decision) and policy (i.e., ADA, Medicaid HCBS) support this movement toward community living. Further, research (e.g., Hewitt et al., 2013a; Nord et al., 2014) demonstrates the positive outcomes of individuals with IDD living in the community.

As individuals with IDD begin to live in the community (Larson, Lakin, & Hill, 2012), the next generation of individuals with IDD and their caregivers may never know or experience institutionalization (Shogren, 2008). As a result, they may be apt to repeat past mistakes (e.g., institutionalization, segregated housing). By having the public—including researchers and practitioners–have a common value about inclusion for all, we can avoid repeating past mistakes.

Implications for Policy. In contrast to the inclusion for all principle, there exists and is support for intentional communities. Indeed, the issues of aging caregivers, an insufficient adult service delivery system, limited access to affordable housing, and waiting lists for services have led some families to explore intentional communities. An intentional community is "a group of people who live together or share common facilities and who regularly associate with each other on the basis of explicit common values" (Fellowship for Intentional Community, 2018, p. 8). Such communities have many forms (e.g., disability specific apartment complexes, farmsteads for people with autism, and gated communities for people with IDD). There are ongoing arguments for and against such communities (see Coalition for Community Choice, 2016 and Autistic Self Advocacy Network, 2015). However, what remains to be seen is the impact of the Centers for Medicare and Medicaid Services Final Settings Rule on the funding of such locations. The Final Rule establishes requirements for Medicaid-funded home and community-based settings that operate under 1915(c), 1915(i), and 1915(k) of the Social Security Act. In addition, the Final Rule excludes certain settings as permissible to provide home and community-based services such as ICFs/ID, nursing facilities, and hospitals. The rule also identifies other settings presumed institutional or that have the effect of isolating individuals from their peers not receiving Medicaid-funded HCBS—this may include intentional communities. If states wish to fund Medicaid-funded services in such settings, the state will need to participate in a "heightened scrutiny" process to determine if such settings are eligible to receive Medicaid-funded HCBS on a case-by-case basis (Centers for Medicare and Medicaid Services, 2014a, 2014b, 2014c).

4.3 The Transdisciplinary Nature of Aging and Disability

Implications for Research and Practice. In line with the graying of America, individuals with IDD are also aging. Specifically, they are outliving their parents for the first time. As a result, families—including parents and siblings–are having longer periods of caregiving (Heller, Caldwell, & Factor, 2007). Notably, however, individuals with IDD also experience an earlier onset of aging-related conditions and worse health (Bittles et al., 2002; Haveman et al., 2010). Because of the longer lives of individuals with IDD and their greater propensity for worse health, it seems prudent to conduct transdisciplinary research and practice between the fields of disability and aging. In this way, disability researchers and practitioners can learn from gerontology research and vice versa. Ultimately, by learning from both fields, the lives of individuals with IDD may be improved.

Unfortunately, little research exists that reflects both the disability and aging fields. As one of the few studies to do this, Heller, Fisher, Marks, and Hsieh (2014) conducted a literature review of health interventions in the fields of disability and aging. They identified five ways each field could learn from one another: use of theory, stronger research designs, use of natural settings, focus on specific diseases or conditions, and use of peer mentors. At the federal level, there are beginning efforts to increase collaboration between disability and aging agencies (Iezzoni, 2014). Future research and practice should continue to reflect this transdisciplinary approach.

Implications for Policy. Increasingly states are implementing managed long-term services and supports (MLTSS) as a means of reducing costs. Within MLTSS programs, states usually contract with managed care organizations (MCOs) to receive a fixed payment; in return, such organizations provide LTSS for individuals within the state (Owen et al., 2015). The goal of MLTSS is to provide more integrated services (i.e., coordination) while also being more efficient. Most states use MLTSS for aging individuals. For example, in March of 2018, 23 states were utilizing MLTSS; however, only eight states included LTSS for people with IDD (Vardaman, 2018).

There exists, however, concern about provision of MLTSS to individuals with IDD as findings regarding service access and care coordination are inconsistent (Williamson et al., 2016) and achievement of cost-savings as a result of MLTSS utilization varies (Libersky, Stepanczuk, Lester, Liao, & Lipson, 2016). Indeed, the President's Committee for People with Intellectual Disabilities (2013) noted that MLTSS is a major concern for individuals with IDD. Thus, moving forward, it is important to consider whether policies, such as MLTSS, may be appropriate and/or need to be revised for aging individuals with IDD.

4.4 Family Advocacy

Implications for Research and Practice. Medicaid HCBS is only one policy impacting adults with IDD and their families. Indeed, there are innumerable other policies which impact adults with IDD (e.g., the ADA, Workforce Innovation and Opportunity Act, Social Security, MFP). In addition to such policies, families also need to stay updated about relevant caselaw that can have sweeping implications on the service delivery system (e.g., *Olmstead*). As such, families—namely parents and siblings—need to learn to navigate such policies to be able to access needed services for their offspring.

To date, there are few interventions designed to increase access to understanding and navigating the adult service delivery system. One such intervention is the Volunteer Advocacy Project-Transition (VAP-T). In this intervention, parents of young adults with autism spectrum disorder (ASD) learn about various service delivery systems and related policies so they can better access services for their offspring (Taylor, Hodapp, Burke, Rabideau, & Waitz-Kudla, 2017). Notably, however, such interventions are often only offered in English and primarily attended by White, well-educated families. Given the service disparities with among minority (versus White) families (Bershadsky et al., 2014; Balcazar et al., 2012), it seems crucial to make such interventions available to minority families.

In addition to learning one's rights and having knowledge about various service delivery systems, families also need the capacity and skills to be able to conduct legislative advocacy. Historically, parent advocacy has come in the form of parent interest groups which reflect grassroots, social movements (e.g., The Arc of the United States, Itkonen, 2009). Given the tremendous potential for drastic changes to current policies, parents need to continue to band together to ensure ongoing funding and monitoring of any changes to the adult service delivery system. Notably, other family members—namely siblings—should also be included in such efforts given their potential roles as the next generation of caregivers.

4.5 Ongoing Co-residence of Adults With IDD and Their Families

Implications for Research and Practice. As noted in this manuscript, many individuals with IDD continue to live with their families well into adulthood thereby elongating the duration of caregiving. To address this, researchers and practitioners should identify the needs of individuals with IDD and their family members who remain in the family home. For example, given the tremendous number of hours dedicated to caregiving (Anderson et al., 2018), researchers may consider developing interventions or supports to alleviate some caregiving duties. Practitioners may offer supports—natural or formal—to best support both the individual with IDD and the family member.

Additionally, researchers and practitioners should recognize the presence of compound caregiving (Perkins, 2010). For example, siblings of adults with IDD are often referred to as the "club sandwich" generation as they may fulfill three simultaneous caregiving roles for their: brother or sister with IDD, aging parent, and own offspring. If the individual with IDD and their own offspring are living in their homes, more support may be needed to alleviate caregiving stress and reduce burden. Additional research is needed to identify the prevalence of compound caregiving with respect to co-residence as well as to determine needed supports and services.

Implications for Policy. Direct support professionals (DSPs) are a critical part of the support system for many individuals with IDD. DSPs assist individuals with IDD in leading self-determined lives by accessing their communities and meeting their physical, personal and household management skills, and developing and maintaining friendships in a person-centered manner (NADSP, 2016). The Bureau of Labor Statistics (2018) reports that the need for home health aides and personal care aides will increase by 41% (n = 1,208,800) in the period between 2016–26, which is more rapid than average in comparison to other industries. Thirty years of low wages, slim benefits, and limited opportunities for career advancement have resulted in high turnover and vacancy rates among DSPs. The demand for DSPs is not currently being met by the numbers entering the workforce and will likely not be met without substantial changes in the recruitment, training, and support of this group (President's Committee for People with Intellectual Disabilities, 2017).

Thus, policy needs to address the issue of DSPs. Specifically, policy should consider mandating a state rate for DSPs that corresponds with a liveable wage. Additionally, all states should consider allowing individuals with IDD to hire their family members as DSPs or personal support workers. Especially in light of the impact of caregiving on financial well-being and the number of hours spent on caregiving, offering financial compensation to family caregivers may alleviate their financial stresses as well as reduce turnover and improve quality. In a previous study wherein siblings could be paid as personal support workers, many siblings reported the importance of having that income (Burke et al., 2015).

4.6 Individuals With IDD Who Do Not Receive Formal Services

Implications for Research and Practice. Despite the growth in the HCBS waiver program and subsequent national public spending on IDD supports and services, in 2016, there were 423,735 individuals with IDD on a waiting list for 1915(c) HCBS waiver programs. In fact, individuals with IDD made up the majority (65%) of those on waiting lists and had an average wait time of 48 months (O'Malley Watts & Musumeci, 2018). Notably, wait times may vary across states.

Little is known about the needs of individuals with IDD who are not in the formal service system. Largely, data sources for national studies are restricted to those in the formal service sector due to the availability of public spending data (e.g., The State of the States in IDD Project), utilization of residential services (e.g., Residential Information Systems Project), and individual outcomes (e.g., National Core Indicators). Notably, in one of few studies about individuals waiting for services, Burke and Heller (2017) found that individuals with IDD who were in poor health, reflected minority backgrounds, and were non-verbal, reported significantly greater unmet support needs. In addition, individuals with younger caregivers and individuals from low-income backgrounds reported greater unmet service needs. Thus, it seems that there are disparities in service needs among individuals waiting for services. More research is needed to determine whether such results generalize to the population; based on such research, supports should be offered to individuals with IDD and their families.

Implications for Policy. The federal Medicaid program is critical to the IDD service delivery system. In FY 2015, Medicaid made up $49.4 billion (76%) of total spending on IDD supports and services in the United States (Braddock, et al., 2017). During FY 2013–15, 41 states and the District of Columbia increased IDD spending. In fact, national spending increased by 4.1% during that period.

Efforts to reduce federal domestic spending through block-granting Medicaid and instituting per-capita caps ultimately failed in 2017, however, Republican House Speaker Paul Ryan (1st – WI) stated that House Republicans intend to re-visit entitlement reform in 2018 (Stein, 2017). Cuts to the Medicaid program will have a substantial impact on people with IDD and their families (The Arc of the United States, 2017). Should states be in a position to see cuts to federal Medicaid funding without subsequent state revenue increases, they may need to make difficult choices to reduce spending such as reduction in enrollment, decreased provider rates, or service cuts (Rudowitz, 2017).

Congress has addressed this looming crisis through passage of the Recognize, Assist, Include, Support, and Engage Family Caregivers Act of 2017 (RAISE Family Caregivers Act, H.R. 3759) which was signed into law on January 22, 2018 by President Trump (P.L. 115 – 119). It directs the Department of Health and Human Services to develop a National Caregiving Strategy to support family caregivers reflecting their diversity of need. While it addresses family caregivers in general, a caregiving family member and a person with a disability are categorically included as members to be appointed to the Family Caregiving Advisory Council that shall be convened to provide recommendations to the Secretary of Health and Human Services.

REFERENCES

Anderson, L., Hewitt, A., Pettingell, S., Lulinski, A., Taylor, M., & Reagan, J. (2018). *Family and individual needs for disability supports (v.2) community report 2017*. Minnesota: Research and Training Center on Community Living, Institute on Community Integration, University of Minnesota.

Arnold, C. K., Heller, T., & Kramer, J. (2012). Support needs of siblings of people with developmental disabilities. *Intellectual and Developmental Disabilities, 50*, 373–382.

Autistic Self Advocacy Network. (December 15, 2015). *Segregated farmsteads in Arizona aren't "community-based" [Web log post]*. Retrieved from: http://autisticadvocacy.org/2015/12/segregated-farmsteads-in-arizona-arent-community-based/.

Balcazar, F. E., Oberoi, A. K., Suarez-Balcazar, Y., & Alvarado, F. (2012). Predictors of outcomes for African Americans in a rehabilitation state agency: Implications for national policy and practice. *Rehabilitation Education, 26*, 43–54.

Balla, D. A. (1976). Relationship of institution size to quality of care: A review of the literature. *American Journal of Mental Deficiency, 81*(2), 117–124.

Bazelon Center for Mental Health Law. (2009). *Still waiting... the unfulfilled promise of Olmstead: A call to action by the Bazelon center for mental health law on the 10th anniversary of the Supreme Court's decision*. Washington, DC: Author.

Becvar, D. S., & Becvar, R. J. (1999). *Systems theory and family therapy: A primer*. University Press of America.

Bittles, A. H., Petterson, B. A., Sullivan, S. G., Hussain, R., Glasson, E. J., & Montgomery, P. D. (2002). The influence of intellectual disability on life expectancy. *Journal of Gerontology Series A: Biological Sciences and Medical Sciences, 57*, M470–M472.

Bjaanes, A. T., & Butler, E. W. (1974). Environmental variation in community care facilities for mentally retarded persons. *American Journal of Mental Deficiency, 78*, 429–439.

Blacher, J. (2001). Transition to adulthood: Mental retardation, families, and culture. *American Journal on Mental Retardation, 106*, 173–188.

Blacher, J., Lopez, S., Shapiro, J., & Fusco, J. (1997). Contributions to depression in Latina mothers with and without children with retardation: Implications for caregiving. *Family Relations, 22*, 325–334.

Blatt, & Kaplan. (1974). *Christmas in purgatory*. Syracuse, NY: Human Policy Press.

Bourke-Taylor, H., Pallant, J. F., Law, M., & Howie, L. (2012). Predicting mental health among mothers of school-aged children with developmental disabilities: The relative contribution of child, maternal and environmental factors. *Research in Developmental Disabilities, 33*, 1732–1740.

Bowey, L., & McGlaughlin, A. (2007). Older carers of adults with a learning disability confront the future: Issues and preferences in planning. *British Journal of Social Work, 37*, 39–54.

Boyd, B. A., & Correa, V. I. (2005). Developing a framework for reducing the cultural clash between African American parents and the special education system. *Multicultural Perspectives, 7*, 3–11.

Braddock, D., Hemp, R., & Rizzolo, M. C. (2003). *State of the states in developmental disabilities project*. Boulder, CO: University of Colorado.

Braddock, D. L., Hemp, R. E., Rizzolo, M. C., Tanis, E. S., Haffer, L., & Wu, J. (2015). *The state of the states in intellectual and developmental disabilities: Emerging from the Great Recession*. Washington, DC: American Association on Intellectual and Developmental Disabilities.

Braddock, D., Hemp, R., Rizzolo, M. C., Coulter, D., Haffer, L., & Thompson, M. (2005). *The state of the states in DD 2005: Preliminary report*. University of Colorado, Department of Psychiatry and Coleman Institute for Cognitive Disabilities.

Braddock, D., Hemp, R., Rizzolo, M. C., Haffer, L., Tanis, E. S., Lulinski, A., & Wu, J. (2013). *State of the states in developmental disabilities 2013: The great recession and its aftermath*. Boulder, CO: University of Colorado and Chicago, IL: University of Illinois at Chicago.

Braddock, D. L., Hemp, R. E., Tanis, E. S., Wu, J., & Haffer, L. (2017). *The state of the states in intellectual and developmental disabilities: 2017*. Washington, DC: American Association on Intellectual and Developmental Disabilities.

Braddock, D., & Parish, S. L. (2002). An institutional history of disability. In D. Braddock (Ed.), *Disability at the dawn of the 21st century and the state of the states* (pp. 3–61). Washington, DC: American Association on Mental Retardation.

Brockley, J. (2004). Rearing the child who never grew: Ideologies of parenting and intellectual disability in American history (130–164). In S. Noll, & J. W. Trent, Jr. (Eds.), *Mental retardation in America: A historical reader*. New York: New York University Press.

Brown, I., Anand, S., Alan-Fung, W. L., Isaacs, B., & Baum, N. (2003). Family quality of life: Canadian results from an international study. *Journal of Developmental and Physical Disabilities, 15*, 207–229.

Bureau of Labor Statistics, U.S. Department of Labor. (2018). *Occupational outlook handbook, home health aides and personal care aides*. Available: https://www.bls.gov/ooh/healthcare/home-health-aides-and-personal-care-aides.htm.

Burke, M. M., Fish, T., & Lawton, K. (2015). A comparative analysis of adult siblings' perceptions towards caregiving. *Intellectual and Developmental Disabilities, 53*, 143–157.

Burke, M. M., & Fujiura, G. (2013). Advantages and disadvantages of using the Survey of Income and Program Participation (SIPP) to examine caregiver health. *International Review of Research in Developmental Disabilities, 45*, 260–276.

Burke, M. M., & Heller, T. (2017). Disparities in unmet service needs among adults with intellectual and developmental disabilities. *Journal of Applied Research in Intellectual Disabilities, 30*, 898–910.

Burke, M. M., Taylor, J. L., Urbano, R., & Hodapp, R. M. (2012). Predictors of future caregiving by adult siblings of individuals with intellectual and developmental disabilities. *American Journal on Intellectual and Developmental Disabilities, 117*, 33–47.

Caldwell, J. (2006). Consumer-directed supports: Economic, health, and social outcomes for families. *Mental Retardation, 44*, 405–417.

Castles, S. (2004). The factors that make and unmake migration policies. *International Migration Review, 38*, 852–884.

Centers for Medicare and Medicaid Services. (2007). *Brief summaries of Medicare & Medicaid, Title XVIII and Title XIX of the social security act*. Retrieved from: http://www.cms.hhs.gov/MedicareProgramRatesStats/downloads/MedicareMedicaidSummaries2007.pdf.

Centers for Medicare and Medicaid Services. (2008). *Medicaid waiver and demonstration list*. Retrieved from: http://www.cms.hhs.gov/MedicaidStWaivProgDemoPGI/MWDL/list.asp?listpage=15.

Centers for Medicare and Medicaid Services. (2014b). *Eligibility*. Retrieved from: http://www.medicaid.gov/Medicaid-CHIP-Program-Information/By-Topics/Eligibility/Eligibility.html.

Centers for Medicare and Medicaid Services. (2014c). *Money follows the person technical assistance*. Retrieved from: http://www.medicaid.gov/State-Resource-Center/Medicaid-State-Technical-Assistance/Money-Follows-the-Person-Tech-Assist/Money-Follows-the-Person-TA.html.

Centers for Medicare and Medicaid Services. (2014a). *Fact sheet: Summary of key provisions of the home and community-based services (HCBS) settings final rule. (CMS 2249-F2296-F)*. Available: https://www.medicaid.gov/medicaid/hcbs/downloads/hcbs-setting-fact-sheet.pdf.

Centers for Medicare and Medicaid Services. (2018a). *Intermediate care facilities for individuals with intellectual disability*. Available: https://www.medicaid.gov/medicaid/ltss/institutional/icfid/index.html.

Centers for Medicare and Medicaid Services. (2018b). *State waivers list*. Retrieved from: https://www.medicaid.gov/medicaid/section-1115-demo/demonstration-and-waiver-list/index.html.

Chen, S. C., Ryan-Henry, S., Heller, T., & Chen, E. H. (2001). Health status of mothers of adults with intellectual disability. *Journal of Intellectual Disability Research: JIDR, 45*, 439–449.

Cicirelli, V. G. (2000). An examination of the trajectory of the adult child's caregiving for an elderly parent. *Federal Register, 49*, 169–175.

Coalition for Community Choice. (February 26, 2016). *Home and community: An individual choice, not an ideological debate [Web log post]*. Retrieved from: http://www.coalitionforcommunitychoice.org/2016/02/home-and-community-an-individual-choice-not-an-ideological-debate/.

Davis, N. O., & Carter, A. S. (2008). Parenting stress in mothers and fathers of toddlers with autism spectrum disorders: Associations with child characteristics. *Journal of Autism and Developmental Disorders, 38*, 1278–1289.

Davys, D., Haigh, C., & Mitchell, D. (2010). Futures planning, parental expectation and sibling concern for people who have a learning disability. *Journal of Intellectual Disabilities, 14*, 167–183.

Department of Health and Human Services. (2015). *Community first choice: Final report to Congress*. Washington, DC: Author.

Emerson, E. (2007). Poverty and people with intellectual disabilities. *Mental Retardation and Developmental Disability Research Reviews, 13*, 107–113.

Engel, J. (2006). *Poor people's medicine: Medicaid and American charity care since 1965*. Durham, NC: Duke University Press.

Erevelles, N., & Minnear, A. (2010). Unspeakable offenses: Untangling race and disability in discourses of intersectionality. *Journal of Literacy and Cultural Disability Studies, 4*, 127–146.

Farber, B. (1968). *Mental Retardation: Its social context and social consequences*. Boston: Houghton Mifflin Company.

Fellowship for Intentional Community. (2018). Retrieve on May 8, 2018 from https://www.ic.org/

Ferguson, P. M. (2004). The legacy of the almshouse. In S. Noll, & J. W. Trent, Jr. (Eds.), *Mental retardation in America: A historical reader*. New York, NY: University Press.

Field, R. (2007). *Health care regulation in America: Complexity, confrontation, and compromise*. Oxford, England: Oxford University Press.

Freedman, R., Krauss, M., & Seltzer, M. (1997). Aging parents' residential plans for adults with mental retardation. *Mental Retardation, 35*, 114–123.

Friedman, C. (2017). A national analysis of Medicaid home and community based services waivers for people with intellectual and developmental disabilities: FY 2015. *Intellectual and Developmental Disabilities, 55*, 281–302.

Fujiura, G. T. (2015). Perspectives on the Publication of Qualitative Research. *Intellectual and developmental disabilities, 53*(5), 323–328.

Gilleard, C. J., Gilleard, E., Gledhill, K., & Whittick, J. (1984). Caring for the elderly mentally infirm at home: A survey of the supporters. *Journal of Epidemiology and Community Health, 38*, 319–325.

Greenberg, J. S., Seltzer, M. M., & Greenley, J. R. (1993). Aging parents of adults with disabilities: The gratifications and frustrations of later-life caregiving. *The Gerontologist, 33*, 542–550.

Grossman, B. R., & Magaña, S. (2016). Introduction to the special issue: Family support of persons with disabilities across the life course. *Journal of Family Social Work, 19*, 237–251.

Haley, W. E., & Perkins, E. A. (2004). Current status and future directions in family caregiving and aging people with intellectual disabilities. *Journal of Policy and Practice in Intellectual Disabilities, 1*, 24–30.

Hanline, M. F., & Daley, S. E. (1992). Family coping strategies and strengths in Hispanic, African-American, and Caucasian families of young children. *Topics in Early Childhood Special Education, 12*, 351–366.

Harry, B. (2002). Collaboration with culturally and linguistically diverse families: Ideal versus reality. *Exceptional Children, 74*, 372–388.

Haveman, M., Heller, T., Lee, L., Maaskant, M., Shooshtari, S., & Strydom, A. (2010). Major health risks in aging persons with intellectual disabilities: An overview of recent studies. *Journal of Policy and Practice in Intellectual Disabilities, 7*, 59–69.

Heller, T. (2002). Residential settings and outcomes for individuals with intellectual disabilities. *Current Opinion in Psychiatry, 15*, 503–508.

Heller, T., & Arnold, C. K. (2010). Siblings of adults with developmental disabilities: Psychosocial outcomes, relationships, and future planning. *Journal of Policy and Practice in Intellectual Disabilities, 7*, 16–25.

Heller, T., Caldwell, J., & Factor, A. (2007). Aging family caregivers: Policies and practices. *Developmental Disabilities Research Reviews, 13*, 136–142.

Heller, T., & Factor, A. (1993). Aging family caregivers: Support resources and changes in burden and placement desire. *American Journal on Mental Retardation, 98*, 417–426.

Heller, T., & Factor, A. (1994). Facilitating future planning and transitions out of the home. In M. M. Seltzer, M. W. Krauss, & M. P. Janicki (Eds.), *Life course perspectives on adulthood and old age* (pp. 39–50). Washington DC: The American Association on Mental Retardation.

Heller, T., Fisher, D., Marks, B., & Hsieh, K. (2014). Interventions to promote health: Crossing networks of intellectual and developmental disabilities and aging. *Disability and Health Journal, 7*, S24–S32.

Heller, T., & Kramer, J. (2009). Involvement of adult siblings of persons with developmental disabilities in future planning. *Intellectual and Developmental Disabilities, 47*, 208–219.

Heller, T., Miller, A. B., & Factor, A. (1997). Adults with mental retardation as supports to their parent: Effects on parental caregiving appraisal. *Mental Retardation, 35*, 338–346.

Hemp, R., & Braddock, D. (2003). *Ten questions: On the role of Medicaid for persons with developmental disabilities in the United States. State of the states in developmental disabilities project.* Department of Psychiatry and Coleman Institute for Cognitive Disabilities, University of Colorado.

Hess, R. S., Molina, A. M., & Kozleski, E. B. (2006). Until somebody hears me: Parent voice and advocacy in special educational decision making. *British Journal of Special Education, 33*, 148–157.

Hewitt, A., Agosta, J., Heller, T., Williams, A. C., & Reinke, J. (2013a). Families of individuals with intellectual and developmental disabilities: Policy, funding, services, and experiences. *Intellectual and Developmental Disabilities, 51*, 349–359.

Hodapp, R. M., Glidden, L. M., & Kaiser, A. P. (2005). Siblings of persons with disabilities: Toward a research agenda. *Mental Retardation, 43*, 334–338.

Holahan, J., & Chen, V. (2011). *Changes in health insurance coverage in the great recession, 2007-2010.* Washington, DC: Kaiser Commission on Medicaid and the Uninsured.

Iezzoni, L. I. (2014). Policy concerns raised by the growing US population aging with disability. *Disability and Health Journal, 7*, 64–68.

Irvin, C. V., Bohl, A., Stewart, K., Williams, S. R., Steiner, Al, Denny-Brown, N., … Peebles, V. (2017). *Money follows the person 2015 annual evaluation report*. Cambridge, MA: Mathematica Policy Research.

Itkonen, T. (2009). *The role of special education interest groups in national policy*. Cambria Press.

Jokinen, N. S., & Brown, R. I. (2011). Family quality of life and older-aged families of adults with an intellectual disability. In R. Kober (Ed.), *Enhancing the quality of life of people with intellectual disabilities: From theory to practice* (pp. 279–303). The Netherlands: Springer.

Jones, K. W. (2004). Education for children with mental retardation: Parent activism, public policy, and family ideology in the 1950s. In S. Noll, & J. W. Trent, Jr. (Eds.), *Mental retardation in America: A historical reader* (pp. 322–350). New York, NY: New York University Press.

Jones, J. L. (2012). Factors associated with self-concept: Adolescents with intellectual disabilities share their perspectives. *Intellectual and Developmental Disabilities, 50*, 31–40.

Kaiser Commission on Medicaid and the Uninsured. (2011). *Update: State budgets in recession and recovery*. Washington, DC: Kaiser Family Foundation.

Kim, S., Larson, S. A., & Lakin, K. C. (1999). Behavioral outcomes of deinstitutionalization for people with intellectual disabilities: A review of studies conducted between 1980 and 1999. In *Policy research brief* (Vol. 10). Minneapolis, MN: University of Minnesota, Institute on Community Integration.

Kozma, A., Mansell, J., & Beadle-Brown, J. (2009). Outcomes in different residential settings for people with intellectual disability: A systematic review. *American Association on Intellectual and Developmental Disabilities, 114*, 193–222.

Krauss, M. W., Seltzer, M. M., & Jacobson, H. T. (2005). Adults with autism living at home or in non-family settings: Positive and negative aspects of residential status. *Journal of Intellectual Disability Research, 49*, 111–124.

Lakin, K. C., Bruininks, R. H., & Sigford, B. B. (1981). Early perspectives on the community adjustment of mentally retarded people. *Monograph of the American Association of Mental Deficiency, 4*, 28–36.

Larson, S. A., Eschenbacher, H. J., Anderson, L. L., Taylor, B., Pettingell, S., Hewitt, A., … Bourne, M. L. (2018). *In-home and residential long-term supports and services for persons with intellectual or developmental disabilities: Status and trends through 2016*. Minneapolis: University of Minnesota, Research and Training Center on Community Living, Institute on Community Integration.

Larson, S. A., & Lakin, K. C. (1989). Deinstitutionalization of persons with mental retardation: Behavioral outcomes. *The Journal of the Association for Persons with Severe Handicaps, 14*, 324–332.

Larson, S. A., Lakin, K. C., & Hill, S. L. (2012). Behavioral outcomes of moving from institutional to community living for people with intellectual and developmental disabilities: US studies from 1977 to 2010. *Research and Practice for Persons with Severe Disabilities, 37*, 1–12.

Lee, C. (2018). *A systematic literature review of future planning among families of individuals with disabilities* (in preparation).

Lee, C., & Burke, M. M. (2018). Caregiving roles of siblings of adults with intellectual and developmental disabilities: A systematic review. *Journal of Policy and Practice in Intellectual Disabilities* (in press).

Libersky, J., Stepanczuk, C., Lester, R., Liao, K., & Lipson, D. (March 2016). *Medicaid managed long-term services and supports: Themes from site visits to five states. Working Paper 44*. Princeton, NJ: Mathematica Policy Research.

Lulinski Norris, A. (2008). *The impact of Medicaid drug policies on people with intellectual and developmental disabilities*. Unpublished Master's thesis. University of Illinois at Chicago.

Magaña, S., & Smith, M. J. (2006a). Health outcomes of midlife and older Latina and Black American mothers of children with developmental disabilities. *Mental Retardation, 44*, 224–234.

Magaña, S., & Smith, M. J. (2006b). Psychological distress and well-being of Latina and non-Latina white mothers of youth and adults with an autism spectrum disorder: Cultural attitudes towards coresidence status. *American Journal of Orthopsychiatry, 76*, 346.

Magaña, S., & Smith, M. J. (2008). Health behaviors, service utilization, and access to care among older mothers of color who have children with developmental disabilities. *Intellectual and Developmental Disabilities, 46*, 267–280.

Mailick Seltzer, M., Greenberg, J. S., Floyd, F. J., Pettee, Y., & Hong, J. (2001). Life course impacts of parenting a child with a disability. *American Journal on Mental Retardation, 106*, 265–286.

Mercadente, M. T., Evans-Lacko, S., & Paula, C. S. (2009). Perspectives of intellectual disability in Latin American countries: Epidemiology, policy, and services for children and adults. *Current Opinion in Psychiatry, 22*, 469–474.

Metzel, D. S. (2004). Historical social geography. In S. Noll, & J. W. Trent, Jr. (Eds.), *Mental retardation in America: A historical reader* (pp. 420–444). New York, NY: New York University Press.

NADSP. (March 2016). *Direct support professional competency areas*. National Alliance of Direct Support Professionals. Available: https://nadsp.org/wp-content/uploads/2017/07/National-Direct-Support-Professional-Competency-Areas-Brochure-FINAL.pdf.

National Alliance for Caregiving and AARP Public Policy Institute. Caregiving in the US. 2015. Retrieved from: http://www.aarp.org/content/dam/aarp/ppi/2015/caregiving-in-the-united-states-2015-report-revised.pdf.

Navaie-Waliser, M., Feldman, P. H., Gould, D. A., Levine, C., Kuerbis, A. N., & Donelan, K. (2002). When the caregiver needs care: The plight of vulnerable caregivers. *American Journal of Public Health, 92*, 409–413.

Ng, T., Wong, A., & Harrington, C. (2012). Olmstead *and* Olmstead *related lawsuits*. Retrieved from: http://www.pascenter.org/olmstead/olmsteadcases.php.

Nord, D., Kang, Y., Ticha, R., Hamre, K., Fay, M., & Mosely, C. (2014). *Residential setting and individual outcomes: An assessment of existing national core Indicators research policy Brief, 24*. Minneapolis, MN: Research and Training Center on Community Living at the University of Minnesota.

Owen, R., Bonardi, A., Bradley, V., Butterworth, J., Caldwell, J., Cooper, R., … Rizzolo, M. K. (2015). Long-term services and supports. *Inclusion, 3*, 233–241.

O'Malley Watts, M., & Musumeci, M. (2018). *Medicaid home and community-based services: Results from a 50-state survey of enrollment, spending, and program policies (Publication #9140)*. Retrieved from The Henry J. Kaiser Family Foundation website: http://files.kff.org/attachment/Report-Medicaid-Home-and-Community-Based-Services.

Pastrana, A. (2004). Black identity constructions: Inserting intersectionality, bisexuality, and Afro-Latinidad into Black studies. *Journal of African American Studies, 8*, 74–89.

Pearlin, L. I., Menaghan, E. G., Lieberman, M. A., & Mullan, J. T. (1981). The stress process. *Journal of Health and Social Behavior, 2*, 337–356.

Perkins, E. A. (2010). The compound caregiver: A case study in multiple caregiving roles. *Clinical Gerontologist, 33*, 248–254.

Perkins, E. A., & Haley, W. E. (2010). Compound caregiving: When lifelong caregivers undertake additional caregiving roles. *Rehabilitation Psychology, 55*, 409–416.

Perkins, E. A., & van Heumen, L. (2016). Parental caregiving and later life planning. In B. S. Nelson Goff, & N. P. Springer (Eds.), *Intellectual and developmental disabilities: A road map for families and professionals*. Routledge/Taylor & Francis.

Pinquart, M., & Sörensen, S. (2007). Correlates of physical health of informal caregivers: A meta-analysis. *The Journals of Gerontology Series B: Psychological Sciences and Social Sciences, 62*, 126–P137.

President's Committee for People with Intellectual Disabilities. (2017). *America's direct support workforce crisis: Effects on people with intellectual disabilities, families, communities, and the U.S. economy*. Washington, DC: Author.

Prouty, R. W., Smith, G., & Lakin, K. C. (2007). *Residential services for persons with developmental disabilities: Status and trends through 2006*. Minneapolis: University of Minnesota, Research and Training Center on Community Living, Institute on Community Integration.

Pruchno, R. A., & McMullen, W. F. (2004). Patterns of service utilization by adults with a developmental disability: Type of service makes a difference. *American Journal on Mental Retardation, 109*, 362–378.

Recognize, assist, include, support, and engage family caregivers act. Public law 115–119.(2017). Available: https://www.congress.gov/bill/115th-congress/house-bill/3759/actions.

Reinhard, S. C., Feinberg, L. F., Choula, R., & Houser, A. (2015). Valuing the invaluable: 2015 update. *Insight on the Issues, 104*, 89–98.

Requirements for states and long term care facilities, 42 C.F.R. § 483.400–480.(1988).

Reynolds, M. C., Gotto, G., Agosta, J., Arnold, K., & Fay, M. L. (2016). *Supporting families across the life course. Critical issues in intellectual and developmental disabilities*. Washington, DC: American Association on Intellectual and Developmental Disabilities.

Rothman, D. J. (1990). *The discovery of the asylum*. New Brunswick, NJ: Aldine Transaction.

Rothman, D. J., & Rothman, S. M. (2005). *The Willowbrook Wars: Bringing the mentally disabled into the community*. New Brunswick: Aldine Transaction.

Rudowitz, R. (2017). *No easy choices: 5 options to respond to per capita caps*. Kaiser Family Foundation. Available: https://www.kff.org/medicaid/issue-brief/no-easy-choices-5-options-to-respond-to-per-capita-caps/.

Rueda, R., Monzo, L., Shapiro, J., Gomez, J., & Blacher, J. (2005). Cultural models of transition: Latina mothers of young adults with developmental disabilities. *Exceptional Children, 71*, 401–414.

Scharlach, A. E., Giunta, N., Chow, J. C. C., & Lehning, A. (2008). Racial and ethnic variations in caregiver service use. *Journal of Aging and Health, 20*, 326–346.

Schulz, R., O'Brien, A. T., Bookwala, J., & Fleissner, K. (1995). Psychiatric and physical morbidity effects of dementia caregiving: Prevalence, correlates, and causes. *The Gerontologist, 35*, 771–791.

Seltzer, G. B. (1981). Community residential adjustment: The relationship among environment, performance, and satisfaction. *American Journal of Mental Deficiency, 85*, 624–630.

Seltzer, M. M., Floyd, F. J., Song, J., Greenberg, J. S., & Hong, J. (2011). Midlife and aging parents of adults with intellectual and developmental disabilities: Impacts of lifelong parenting. *American Journal on Intellectual and Developmental Disabilities, 116*, 479–499.

Seltzer, M. M., & Krauss, M. W. (1994). Aging parents who co-reside with adult children. The impact of lifelong caregiving. In M. M. Seltzer, M. W. Krauss, & M. P. Janicki (Eds.), *Life-course perspectives on adulthood and old age* (pp. 3–18). Washington, DC: American Association on Mental Retardation.

Shogren, K. A. (2008). Leadership in the field of intellectual and developmental disabilities. *Intellectual and Developmental Disabilities, 46*, 393–395.

Smith, G. C., Tobin, S. S., & Fullmer, E. M. (1995). Elderly mothers caring at home for offspring with mental retardation: A model of permanency planning. *American Journal on Mental Retardation, 99*, 487–499.

Stein, J. (December 6, 2017). Ryan says Republicans to target welfare, Medicare, Medicaid spending in 2018. *The Washington Post*. Available: https://www.washingtonpost.com/news/wonk/wp/2017/12/01/gop-eyes-post-tax-cut-changes-to-welfare-medicare-and-social-security/?utm_term=.1802d2ff075b.

Steinglass, P. (1987). A systems view of family interaction and psychopathology. In T. Jacob (Ed.), *Family interaction and psychopathology* (pp. 25–66). New York, NY: Plenum Press.

Taylor, J. L., Hodapp, R. M., Burke, M. M., Rabideau, C., & Waitz-Kudla, S. N. (2017). Training parents of youth with autism spectrum disorders to advocate for adult disability services: Results from a pilot randomized controlled trial. *Journal of Autism and Developmental Disorders, 47*, 846–857.

The Arc of the United States. (2017). *The outlook for Medicaid in 2017: Facing cuts, block grants or per capita caps?*. Retrieved: https://www.thearc.org/document.doc?id=5609.

The President's Panel on Mental Retardation. (October 1962). *A proposed program for national action to combat mental retardation*. Author.

Thompson, D., & Wright, S. (2001). *Misplaced and forgotten: People with learning disabilities in residential services for older people*. London: The Foundation for People with Learning Disabilities.

Trent, J. W. (1994). *Inventing the feeble mind: A history of mental retardation in the United States*. Berkeley, CA: University of California Press.

Turnbull, A. P., Turbiville, V., & Turnbull, H. R. (2000). Evolution of family-professional partnerships: Collective empowerment as the model for the early twenty-first century. *Handbook of Early Childhood Intervention, 2*, 630–650.

Turnbull, A. P., & Turnbull, R. (2006). Self-determination: Is a rose by any other name still a rose? Research and Practice for Persons with Severe Disabilities. *31*, 83–88.

U.S. Department of Health and Human Services, 2000.

U.S. Department of Health, Education, and Welfare. (September 1972). *Mental retardation source book of the DHEW*. Washington, DC: Author.

Vardaman, K. (March 1, 2018). *Tailoring MLTSS programs for individuals with intellectual and developmental disabilities*. Medicaid and CHIP Payment and Access Commission. Available: https://www.macpac.gov/wp-content/uploads/2018/03/Tailoring-MLTSS-Programs-for-Individuals-with-Intellectual-and-Developmental-Disabilities.pdf.

Von Bertalanffy, L. (1969). General systems theory and psychiatry—an overview. *General Systems Theory and Psychiatry, 2*, 33–46.

Werner, S., Edwards, M., & Baum, N. (2009). Family quality of life before and after out-of-home placement of a family member with an intellectual disability. *Journal of Policy and Practice in Intellectual Disabilities, 6*, 32–39.

Whitchurch, G. G., & Constantine, L. L. (1993). Systems theory. In P. G. Boss, W. J. Doherty, R. LaRossa, W. R. Schumm, & S. K. Steinmetz (Eds.), *Sourcebook of family theories and methods: A contextual approach* (pp. 325–352). New York: Plenum Press.

Wilgosh, L., Sobsey, D., & Scorgie, K. (2003). *Cultural constructions of families of children with disabilities*. Retrieved from: http://www.arts.ualberta.ca/cms/wilgosh.pdf.

Williams, E. R. (2007). Unnecessary and unjustified: African-American parental perceptions of special education. In *The educational forum* (Vol. 71, No. 3, pp. 250–261). Taylor & Francis Group.

Williamson, H. J., & Perkins, E. A. (2014). Family caregivers of adults with intellectual and developmental disabilities: Outcomes associated with U.S. Services and Supports. *Intellectual and Developmental Disabilities, 52*, 147–159.

Williamson, H. J., Perkins, E. A., Acosta, A., Fitzgerald, M., Agrawal, J., & Massey, O. T. (2016). Family caregivers of individuals with intellectual and developmental disabilities: Experiences with Medicaid managed care long-term services and supports in the United States. *Journal of Policy and Practice in Intellectual Disabilities, 13*, 287–296.

Wolfensberger, W. (1975). The evolution of institutional models in the United States. In *The origin and nature of our institutional models* (Rev. ed., pp. 23–56). Syracuse, NY: Human Policy Press.

Yamaki, K., Hsieh, K., & Heller, T. (2009). Health profile of aging family caregivers supporting adults with intellectual and developmental disabilities at home. *Intellectual and Developmental Disabilities, 47*(6), 425–435.

Zenderland, L. (2004). The parable of the Kallikak family: Explaining the meaning of heredity in 1912. In S. Noll, & J. W. Trent, Jr. (Eds.), *Mental retardation in America: A historical reader* (pp. 165–185). New York, NY: New York University Press.

CHAPTER SIX

Reconceptualizing Natural Supports for People With Disabilities and Their Families

Michelle C. Reynolds*, Susan B. Palmer[§,1] and George S. Gotto*
*University of Missouri at Kansas City - Institute for Human Development, Kansas City, MO, United States
[§]Beach Center on Disability, KUCDD, University of Kansas, Lawrence, KS, United States
[1]Corresponding Author: Email: spalmer@ku.edu

Contents

Abstract

People with intellectual and developmental disabilities (IDD) use natural supports and sometimes receive paid or formal supports in addition to the support families provide. Yet, most of the emphasis of funding and research in our field is on eligibility-specific supports for people with IDD with tangential acknowledgement of families. This

International Review of Research in Developmental Disabilities, Volume 54
ISSN 2211-6095
https://doi.org/10.1016/bs.irrdd.2018.07.006

chapter proposes that to best support people with disabilities and their families, supports should be a logical and efficient integration of all available supports, as opposed to a dichotomy of only two options – paid (eligibility-specific supports) and natural. We explore the historical and theoretical status of integrated supports, especially focusing on the expanded emphasis on natural supports that has evolved within the paradigm of the Charting the LifeCourse framework (Reynolds, St. John, & Gotto, 2012). This framework addresses self- and family-identified strengths and needs for individuals with IDD and their families. It recognizes that individuals with IDD and their families are rooted in social relationships and bureaucratic systems that influence the trajectory of individuals and their families. We suggest that formal supports can enhance natural or informal supports by (a) recognizing and enhancing a person's capacities, (b) strengthening and connecting social networks, (c) leveraging resources within environments accessed by all citizens, and (d) utilizing technological innovations so people with IDD can achieve their preferred quality of life.

1. UNDERSTANDING NATURAL SUPPORTS

Everyone in the world uses supports – whether or not one has a disability. Supports are resources and strategies that enhance human functioning (Luckasson et al., 2002; Thompson et al., 2009). When supports are matched with the strengths and needs of a person, these can enhance the quality of life of individuals (Buntinx & Schalock, 2010), both with and without disabilities.

In the field of disability, the term *natural supports* is a broad descriptor for unpaid or informal supports, rather than being specifically defined (Duggan & Linehan, 2013). Formal supports are usually government-funded, as compared to informal or natural supports not necessarily funded - but facilitated within the community to encourage full participation. To move from a support paradigm with an already-defined array of services to the more individualized process of supporting the person and their families, one must collectively take into account a person with IDD and their family's unique strengths and needs. This change in perspective recognizes the person with disabilities embedded within their family system and within the community that they live (Amado, Stancliffe, McCarron, & McCallion, 2013). In order to support a person and their family to build on strengths, meet established needs, and build a good life within their culture and community, we must rethink the concept of supports and their use beyond formal service systems.

Very few families and people with IDD exclusively receive paid or eligibility-specific supports. Only about 25% of the population of people with developmental disabilities receive funding from the state developmental disability service system, with 58% of this number living in the home of a family member (Larson et al., 2017). Hewitt (2014) confirms that the majority of people with IDD are living with their families, not receiving Medicaid-funded long-term services and supports, and are unknown to state developmental disability agencies. But many people with disabilities, families, professionals, and policy makers assume that people need to have, advocate for, and receive funded services even when these services are less available to families and others in need. Some services are less comprehensive and cover limited needs. For example, Friedman and Spassiani (2017) report that since only $447.5 million in 2014's Medicaid 1915(c) HSBS waiver dollars supported only the initial transition to community living, there remained a need to use natural supports and enhance skills to maintain life in the community long-term. In contrast, *community integration services* (beyond initial transition to the community) were sometimes available as a waiver service using some natural supports to help with adjustment to different living settings, community skill development, problem solving, and/or developing social skills, but these needed to be unique from other services such as residential or day habilitation services (Friedman & Spassiani, 2017). Historically, the primary perspective in the field of disability addressed supports primarily as paid or government-funded programs, which were much less flexible in meeting the overall expressed needs of people with IDD. Nevertheless, in reality, families and people with disabilities may benefit from natural or informal supports in ways beyond the scope of the current focus on formalized systems and services, waiting lists, and shrinking funds throughout the United States.

This chapter will explore the status of integrated supports, especially focusing on the expanded discussion of natural supports that has evolved within the paradigm of the Charting the LifeCourse framework (Reynolds, St. John, & Gotto, 2012) that addresses self- and family-identified strengths and needs for individuals with IDD and their families. After reviewing the history of supports for families and people with IDD, we will describe the content and application of the Charting the LifeCourse framework for families and family members with IDD that reframes the concept of natural supports and extends the characterization of integrated supports to focus on the person and their family as a catalyst for change. Using a holistic person-centered approach, Charting the LifeCourse framework binds informal and relevant formal supports to benefit multiple aspects and life stages of an individual with IDD and their family and friends in the context of home and community over the life span. Finally, we propose a new and more applicable conceptualization of overall supports that characterize the current state of community involvement that is more than social inclusion — a sense of full citizenship for people with disabilities and their families is on the horizon.

Within this chapter, we use the term Intellectual and Developmental Disabilities (IDD), to focus on the need for broader and more self-generated integrated supports to help identify and assist people with more than usual support needs (Brown, Wehmeyer, & Shogren, 2017b). Some people with IDD also could experience Intellectual Disability (ID), a significant limitation in both intellectual functioning and adaptive behavior (some social and/or practical skills) identified prior to age 18 years (Schalock et al., 2010). Developmental Disabilities (DD), as specified by the Developmental Disabilities legislation of 2000 (Developmental Disabilities Assistance and Bill of Rights Amendments of 2000, PL 106-402, 45 CFR 1385.3), has a slightly different meaning. DD includes both cognitive and physical limitations manifested before age 22, with limitations in three of the following: capacity for independent living, economic self-sufficiency, learning, mobility, receptive and expressive language, self-care, and self-direction. The combined term, Intellectual and Developmental Disabilities, includes and better describes the majority of the population of individuals with needs that involve cognitive, physical, and limitations in daily living who need additional services. The construct of IDD also conveys information regarding the ongoing need for supporting the quality of life of the person with IDD within the context of their family and the community in which they live.

2. HISTORY AND CONTEXT OF NATURAL SUPPORTS

According to Wehmeyer, Bersani, and Gagne (2000), three distinct waves characterize how disability was interpreted over time: 1) professionals dominated disability until around 1950 when … 2) families were more likely to assume a role to represent their sons and daughters, followed by, 3) self-advocacy and self-determination which began to emerge about 1970 and continue to the present day. Throughout these waves of historical significance, the supports paradigm has gained an increasing amount of traction to encourage an ever-increasing amount of community inclusion for individuals with IDD.

2.1 Evolution of Supports for People With IDD

Individuals with IDD have a number of experiences and participate in events throughout their lives that involve their related family members, other people who they consider part of their family, the places in which they live, and the larger community. State and national policies not only influence formal services and supports, but these entities might also indirectly impact accessing informal or natural supports to address day-to-day living situations or decision making by people with IDD or decisions made on their behalf. Currently, individuals with IDD make more choices and decisions within their lives, but in the past, disability equated with pathology where professionals spent more time describing impairments and limitations of human functioning rather than understanding individual needs for support (Buntinx, 2013).

Initially, the purpose of creating large congregate settings or institutions was to protect individuals from society in order to keep them safe, but in the early 1900's this aim changed to protecting society from the feebleminded considered to be different at that time (Smith & Wehmeyer, 2012). Individuals with IDD were deemed safer in institutions, but in reality they were subjected to a variety of threats to their well-being including isolation from families, segregation from the community, disease, restriction of personal freedoms, and sometimes, sterilization. Another aspect of the restricted life of a person with IDD was legislation to limit the procreation of people with disabilities through eugenics (Noll, Smith, & Wehmeyer, 2013) or the involuntary sterilization of people with IDD. Instead of supporting basic needs of people with IDD, it brought more restrictions and limitations to the lives of people in institutions. "People with disabilities were looked upon as eternal children, remaining chaste and innocent throughout their lives" (Klein & Strully, 2000, p.167).

Brown, Radford, and Wehmeyer (2017a) mention that "No single event marked the end of the institutional era" (p.30). In general, a constellation of factors such as overcrowding and reduced public interest and funding along with the realization of inequality and human rights violations related to use of drugs, failure of eugenics, and research conducted without consent contributed to the disfavor of institutions as placement for individuals with IDD. Not only did parent and advocacy groups argue for resources to provide care and support in community settings, but professionals in academia and from government agencies continue to work to close institutions in the present day (Brown et al., 2017a).

The Civil Rights era in the United States influenced the self-advocacy movement that began in the late 1970's. According to Ferguson, Ferguson, and Wehmeyer (2013) "a small group of people with ID in Salem, Oregon formulated the phrase "We are people first" (p. 238). Across the United

States, informal self-advocacy groups formed to reaffirm rights and influence families, policy makers, and professionals. Self-Advocates identified with and began to drive the agenda that (a) people with IDD have capacity to make choices and decisions to impact their own lives, (b) can determine a self-selected quality of life, and (c) can live and work in the community, using a desired level of supports and services within their friends and family.

Currently, people with disabilities want services that help them live and participate fully in their community; and they want to have control over how, where, and when those services are provided (Tichá, Hewitt, Nord, & Larson, 2013). Supported Decision Making (SDM; Dinerstein, 2012) is gaining traction in many states to take the place of the somewhat automatic process of establishing guardianship, as youth with IDD become adults. "At the heart of issue are assumptions about the capacity of individuals with disabilities" (Jameson et al., 2015, p. 1) - that people with disabilities are deficient decision-makers. Results of a survey by Jameson and colleagues to investigate guardianship found that professionals involved in transition to adulthood - primarily school personnel - needed more training and comprehension of what imposing guardianship on individuals with disabilities at age 18 implies. This legal mechanism abrogates rights, self-determination, and other important decisions for people with disabilities to others who may or may not have the best interests of a person in mind. Individuals with IDD are often capable of making all or most of the decisions within their lives, with supports provided by people they choose to help them, who know them well, just as this is true for people without disabilities. More research may determine the impact of various models of SDM on the self-determination and quality of life of people with disabilities who exercise more control over the decisions in their lives. However, it is important to acknowledge the need for natural supports in the life of a person with IDD rather than having a system or service or situation imposed upon them by another person, namely their guardian who is not legally required to consult with the person with IDD (Jameson et al., 2015).

In the current strengths-based or social model of disability (Buntinx, 2013), using the lens of positive psychology, disability is seen as less pathological - more affiliated with optimism, hope, and problem solving (Wehmeyer, 2013). This change in disability awareness is encouraging, but people with disabilities and their families must continue to advocate for their desired quality of life to facilitate living, loving, working, and playing in their community. People with IDD should be able to "live

Table 1 Evolution of Elements of Support for Individuals and Families

	Person within Service System and Community	**Family Supports/ Supporting Families**
Before 1950	1700 - 1800, people with disabilities sent to almshouses with inhuman conditions. 1907 - 1958 Eugenics accepted practice Institutionalization is common	Families encouraged to use out of home placement for son/daughter National organizations founded by parents in 1949 The Arc of the US and United Cerebral Policy ***IDD Descriptors: feebleminded, idiocy, mental deficiency***
1950 - 1999	Deinstitutionalization Residential services programs Some social inclusion Medicaid 1965; Guardianship common Normalization –1970's; Self-Advocacy Movement Home and Community Based Waiver 1981; Rehab Act; Education for All Children; IDEA; ADA- 1990	Parent-Family Movement Established education programs outside of public school pre-1975 Education for All children enacted Family Advocacy Family Support Programs (need to look at ADD funded PNS projects) ***IDD Descriptor: Mental Retardation***
2000 - Present	Person-Centered Planning Managed Care Affordable Care Act; Home ownership ADA/Olmsted decision Self-Directed Supports Supported Decision Making Community-Based Settings Rule; (WIOA) Employment First	Sibling movement Family-professional partnerships Voucher programs; Supported Decision Making in lieu of Guardianship Wingspread Conference on Supporting Families *National Community of Practice* ***Descriptors: ID, DD, IDD***

freely within communities of their choosing [with] psychological and social acceptance, and life patterns comparable to people who do not have disability labels" (Rich, 2015, p.37) (Table 1).

2.2 Evolution of the Role of Families and Supports

The shift to understanding disability from a positive perspective, enhanced recognition that parents and caregivers needed services and supports that would enable them to successfully raise their family member at home (Amado et al., 2013) or in a place nearby of one's choosing, rather than in a controlled medical or institutional setting. One of the current National Goals for Families (Reynolds et al., 2015) is to extend understanding of the experiences of individuals with IDD within families and communities outside the purview of IDD systems. People with IDD are still part of their own families, even if individuals live apart from their closest relatives. Thus, even though a person with IDD may receive some formal supports, they also are part of the community in which they and their family live, work, and engage in leisure activities.

2.2.1 History of Supporting Families Movement

Prior to 1950, professionals counseled families to institutionalize their children with IDD (Turnbull & Turnbull, 2000). But, the parent movement that began in 1950 with the formation of the National Association of Parents and Friends of Mentally Retarded Children (later, The Arc of the United States) coincided with a decline in institutional placements and increase in community supports and legislation to support people with IDD. Families challenged the status of current services, education models, legislation, and overall funding for services to support their sons and daughters with IDD (Wehmeyer & Schalock, 2013). Families began to advocate for their sons and daughters with IDD to live at home and go to school like their siblings or peers. As parent advocacy grew over time, individuals with IDD also began to advocate for their own rights, responsibilities, and inclusion in the community. Although we think of self-advocacy as an independent action by individuals with IDD, most self-advocates have the support, encouragement, and appreciation of family and friends in their communities.

By 2000, family support could be characterized by several themes: 1) the nature of family support (cash or vouchers to give families a degree of choice), 2) the extent of family support (services beginning to be less dominated by professionals with more guidance by families), and 3) the place supports were provided (family home and the community). A wide range of government programs existed and families could integrate formal and informal supports, but there was less encouragement to use natural supports outside of the family home (Turnbull & Turnbull, 2000). Some families accessed voucher systems to fund individualized supports and services to promote community living, but the voucher process was cumbersome and limited by bureaucracy.

In the spring of 2011, a group of self-advocates, family members, and professionals developed a National Agenda for Supporting Families at the

Wingspread Conference Center in Racine, Wisconsin. This group acknowledged the need for a continuing effort by families, professionals, and agencies at all levels of impact to engage in perspective taking by supporting families to be valued, respected, and be an essential part of the circle surrounding and encouraging an individual with disabilities (Hecht, Reynolds, Agosta, & McGinley, 2011). The Wingspread discussions generated recommendations for policy and practice such as stable, coordinated, and flexible funding streams for services provided through local, state, and national levels that bridge the gap between natural and formal supports for families and individuals with IDD. Following Wingspread the term, *Supporting families,* replaced the typical *family support* services to emphasize how families can maximize their capacity, strengths, and unique abilities to support their family members with IDD by integrating services and natural supports (Reynolds, 2015).

2.2.2 Natural Supports and Family

In recent years, states have begun to recognize the significant role of families in the lives of people with disabilities. Currently, service systems are focusing more on community supports, and less on settings that isolate and segregate (Dinerstein, 2016). Approximately 18.2% of the entire US population is providing supports to a family member with a disability, chronic illness, or a person who is aging (National Alliance for Caregiving, 2015). These families reported providing 24.4 h of care weekly with 23% of family caregivers providing 40 or more hours per week. Family members that provide day-to-day and long-term supports to members with disabilities are a critical part of the overall system of long-term care for people of any age with any disability and this family contribution is reflected more in federal and state policy. However, it is critical for service systems to view the role of family members and the importance of natural supports, as a way to enhance quality of life instead of only being a financial advantage.

Families, often the primary support for persons with IDD, are tasked with structuring the environment of their son, daughter, sister, brother or unrelated friend to live in the community with little help from federal or state funding. This is also the task of any family — to support members within their circle of influence. However, for people with disabilities there are physical, logistical, and financial differences that could extend beyond typical family roles as their children age. As stated previously approximately 75% of people with IDD do not receive paid or eligibility-specific supports and are entirely dependent on informal supports facilitated by their family.

Consequently, there is a need for supporting families in their role to enhance and engage in natural supports for their loved one with IDD.

One way for a person with IDD to actively engage in planning for current and future needs is for families and professionals to ensure individuals with disabilities are at the center of a plan for living, loving, working, and playing in their community. Person-centered planning (PCP) "is an approach to planning supports that aims to redistribute power from the service system to individuals with IDD and natural supports, improve relationships, and build community" (Martin, Grandia, Ouellette-Kuntz, & Cobigo, 2016, p. 552). Not only is the process important for individuals, but it also involves families in identifying and exploring natural supports within the planning team to meet the identified needs of a person with IDD.

One of the first papers on PCP introduced in the 1980's, described The McGill Action Planning System (Vandercook, York, & Forest, 1989). More recently, MAPs and PATH (O'Brien & Pearpoint, 2002), use visual representations to make the process and outcomes transparent for all. Much the same as the Charting the LifeCourse trajectory and goals planning process, PCP is a way to collaborate, individualize goals, and focus goals on community living activities (Claes, Van Hove, Vandevelde, van Loon, & Schalock, 2010). In either the MAPs or PATH process, a collaborative team of the person with IDD, family members who are invited by their family member with disabilities, service providers (if the person gets paid or unpaid supports), and community members gather to talk about possible goals for the person with IDD. This team can listen and learn a person's story, their dreams, and the person's gifts. It is also important to come up with next steps for achieving a particular goal to support the vision of the person with IDD. Often, the team starts to build a community map, develops action statements, and assigns responsibilities related to a central goal.

A qualitative study of PCP concluded that it is important for the right people to be involved in planning, that attitudes and actions of any provider agencies involved in the planning should be positive, and the disability services system and social environment in the community should be compatible (Bailey & Nixon, 2014; Martin et al., 2016). Beyond this guidance, the involvement of family members is critical to any plan's success. Identifying effective people (who know the person well and are good collaborators), who have the right attitudes (to empower a person with IDD), using the right actions (communication and documentation), is part of effective PCP.

Community living and participation is fundamentally about having the opportunity to make choices about where to live, where or whether to work, with whom to socialize, and other aspects of daily living (Hewitt, 2014). Families of people with IDD facilitate natural supports for community living, either through providing support in their own home or by encouraging people with IDD living elsewhere to use a mix of formal and informal or integrated supports (if they qualify for any paid services), or by combining a variety of natural or informal supports available to all people. Even though a person with IDD may receive some formal supports, they also are part of the community in which they and their family live, work, and engage in leisure activities.

Families play a key role in building social capital (Gotto, Calkins, Jackson, Walker, & Beckman, 2010) for all members including people with IDD. Social capital is a set of relationships and social structures based on trust and reciprocity that develop over time. As suggested by Palmer and Turnbull (2012), "Family participation in the lives of their family member who are initially developing social capital is very important, and is especially critical in connecting individuals with disabilities to existing groups and social structure within smaller communities and the larger world" (p. 17). Families, including siblings and others, are also important facilitators of building self-determination abilities for people with IDD in their family. Families set the stage, maintain particular social and cultural parameters, and promote choice, decision-making, problem solving, goal setting, and self-regulation strategies by providing opportunities and embed ways to build and use abilities in these elements to act as a causal agent in one's life, making choice and decision free of undue influence, and of course, within the framework of one's family culture and needs (Palmer, 2010; Wehmeyer, 1999).

3. A FRAMEWORK FOR INTEGRATING SUPPORTS

3.1 Development of Charting the LifeCourse Framework

The Charting the LifeCourse framework (http://www.lifecoursetools.com/principles/, 2017) evolved within a collaborative process led by Dr. Michelle Reynolds at the Institute for Human Development at the University of Missouri – Kansas City, a University Center for Excellence (UCEDD) in partnership with national and statewide stakeholders (Reynolds et al., 2012). The idea for this framework began to emerge in 2011 and supporting families became the guiding principle of the National Community of Practice on Supporting Families of Individuals with Intellectual and Developmental

Disabilities (CoP), a collaboration with National Association of State Directors of Developmental Disabilities Services. Dr. Reynolds, a family member whose brother experiences IDD, proposed the framework along with her team including Jane St John, the mother of a son who also experiences disabilities. Over a three-year period, the guiding principles and tools evolved utilizing an iterative process driven by self-advocates, family leaders and professional members of the Missouri Family-to-Family Stakeholders group that met at least quarterly. Members of the national CoP including representatives from self-advocate and family networks; developmental disability councils; state developmental disability agencies; education and early childhood departments; and aging and employment services helped to further refine the framework Thus, the Charting the LifeCourse framework is an authentic grassroots activity, informed by personal and others' experiences as family members and self-advocates. These stakeholders saw the need to focus on the individual with IDD within their family to bring about real change and redirection of resources with families in mind. Using the state of Missouri as a launching location, Charting the LifeCourse is now being used in 17 states in a community of practice format, to bring about change at the individual, family, practitioner, and policy levels (Reynolds & Kardell, 2017).

3.2 Theories That Drive the Framework

The Charting the LifeCourse framework supports individuals within their family to benefit from integrated supports and services. Family systems theory (Bowen & Kerr, 1988) recognizes that the family plays a key role in both emotional and physical well-being across the life course since most individuals have contact with their family of origin through their entire lives. Families often influence day-to-day lives; families come together to both celebrate and help each other through crises. Family systems theory emphasizes the idea that families are continuous entities, with rules, beliefs, and values that shape members over time. A family systems framework influences professionals to not only support the individual with IDD, but also to focus on the family as a whole while acknowledging the many sub-systems within a family that emphasize family interaction (Turnbull, Turnbull, Erwin, Soodak, & Shogren, 2015). Family dynamics (e.g. structures, roles, communication patterns, boundaries, and power relations) impact human relationships, such as what draws people together, drives them apart, and any conflict and intergenerational transmission (Rothbaum, Rosen, Ujiie, & Uchida, 2002). Family functions change over time but could include daily care of a family member with disabilities, community involvement and advocacy, economic support or guidance for any members, and spiritual and social encouragement, to illustrate a few of the endless possibilities that depend on individual and family preferences, interests, and resources (Turnbull et al., 2015).

At a basic level of meeting identified needs, Charting the LifeCourse framework fulfills a hierarchy of needs similar to that of Maslow (1970). Maslow's theory of motivation details how individuals are uniquely qualified experts and competent resources in their own health and healing in medical and other contexts (Zalenski & Raspa, 2006). Maslow's theory explains human motivation based on a hierarchy of five basic needs: Physiological (food, water, and shelter), Safety (physical and mental safety and stability), Love/Belonging (relationships and belonging), Esteem (being respected or valued), and Self-actualization (reaching full potential). Beyond the need for meeting biological functions (physiological needs), Safety of one's body, resources, family, health, and/or property is very important. Maslow lists Love/Belonging as a higher-level need for friendship, family, and intimacy followed by Esteem (both self-esteem and that of others related to one's confidence and achievement). The highest level of achievement of needs is that of Self-Actualization which involves morality, creativity, spontaneity, problem solving and other higher-level needs related to people functioning in home and community settings. According to Maslow's theory, people reach an optimal level of functioning when their deficiency (safety needs, love/belonging needs) *and* growth needs (Esteem and Self-Actualization) are met (Noltemeyer, Bush, Partton, & Bergen, 2012). Maslow's theory "identified several universal requirements for human growth and development, and it posits that certain needs take precedence over others" (Duncan & Blugis, 2011, p. 326). In like fashion the Charting the LifeCourse framework provides a pathway to explore unmet needs through a method of determining one's vision for the future and current trajectory for addressing immediate integrated supports and services. In addition, the LifeCourse framework supplies a model for people with IDD and their families to self-identify (a) integrated supports, (b) how professionals can best assist on a person-by-person basis, and (c) informs policy makers and people within systems initiatives to supports that are flexible enough to meet individual needs.

Using a Life Course Theory perspective, Charting the LifeCourse framework addresses a way to impact and influence the trajectory or pathway of a person with IDD and their family at different ages and stages, meeting identified needs. Elder (1998) suggests looking at how something works throughout life may spark thinking about "social change, life pathways, and individual development as modes of continuity and change" (p. 1). The Charting the LifeCourse framework addresses the present needs, but also addresses previous stages and what actions lead to future outcomes. Families can support a person with disabilities to promote good lives by anticipating and addressing current needs of their family members with IDD with the future in mind. Life Course Theory addresses multiple transitions that involve changes in life status or roles, entrance or departure of friends and family members, or a life stage. Hutchinson (2015) mentions trajectories as encompassing multiple transitions throughout life. Transitions are the stage-like changes in roles and statuses that differ from previous roles in a person's life, but usually represent a discrete time, rather than a continuous track. In contrast, trajectories are a long-term pattern of stability and change that might include one or more transitional events (Elder, Johnson, & Crosnoe, 2003). A primary part of person-centered planning using Charting the LifeCourse includes determining a trajectory that supports positive life experiences, while determining what negative events could interfere. Since the Charting the LifeCourse framework is designed to be used in multiple life stages (prenatal/infancy, early childhood, school age, transition, adulthood, and aging/end of life) it exemplifies life course theory and brings this concept into practice.

Socio-ecological theory is based on person-environmental fit, in which the individual is rooted in social relationships that influence the life-span trajectory (Hurst, Ramsdell, & Sorice, 2017). Each and every person lives in an environment that is akin to themselves, within connections that involve family, friends, and acquaintances that are nested within a community which is guided by the government and leadership of others for whom we vote. Bronfenbrenner's (1989) model of environmental organization addresses the qualities and immediate environment of any person and how this and other enveloping levels of the environment might influence growth and development over time. The socioecological model guides our thinking that people with disabilities can successfully adjust to their environment, by determining needs, intensity of supports, and rooting themselves in social relationships (natural supports) that enhance human functioning (Buntinx & Schalock, 2010; Thompson et al., 2009).

The Charting the LifeCourse framework also addresses the constructs of Self- Determination and Quality of Life. Self-determination involves acting as a causal agent in one's life, using volitional action to make choices and decisions that affect one's quality of life (Wehmeyer et al., 2007). Self-determination does not mean that people must act without support or that self-determination is an actual service or option to enhance one's life. Rather, we need to see people acting in a self-determined manner to make choices and decisions, solve problems, and meet self-selected goals. Causal Agency Theory (Shogren et al., 2015) combines earlier understanding of self-determination and motivational theories to explain how self-determination changes over time. Within Causal Agency Theory, Shogren and colleagues describe a self-determined individual as making continuous choices and displaying self-determined actions based on personal preferences as volitional action. In addition, *agentic action,* a second element of this theory, describes the pathways, self-direction, and goal setting and attainment skills. Agentic action is analogous to the short-term trajectory activity within the Charting the LifeCourse framework that identifies actions to take for goal completion. The third element of Causal Agency Theory is action-control beliefs, the self-awareness or self-knowledge needed to take actions to meet a goal or achieve a desired outcome. Self-determination develops over the lifespan as an individual grows, changes, becomes more competent, and is able to express their needs, solve problems, makes decisions, and become more self-aware to achieve their self-identified quality of life (Palmer, 2010).

The construct of Quality of Life is explained by a set of core domains organized into three factors of well-being (emotional, material, physical); independence (personal development), self-determination, and social participation (interpersonal relations, social inclusion, and rights) representing the needs of individuals (Schalock, 2000). There is a positive relationship between self-determination and a higher quality of life (Lachapelle et al.,2005; Wehmeyer & Schwartz, 1998). The field is also recognizing the need for social capital, relationships, and the importance of the context of the family. Building on the concept of individual quality of life, Family Quality of Life (FQOL) is defined by conditions in which the family's needs are met, they are able to enjoy their time together, and family members have the opportunity to engage in activities that are important to them (Park et al., 2003). Over the past 25 years, FQOL has become a valued outcome of policies and services (Dunst & Bruder, 2002; Summers et al., 2005; Turnbull, Brown, & Turnbull, 2004). FQOL is considered a natural extension of individual quality of life and takes into account what all family members need to have a good life (Poston et al., 2003); however, quality of life is not often considered in service delivery. The choices individuals make in different life domain areas (e.g. meaningful day activities, employment, community living, safety/security, healthy living, social and spirituality, and citizenship and advocacy) impact their quality of life and that of their entire family system.

3.3 Principles of Charting the LifeCourse Framework

In recognition that families have significant needs that often go unmet, the Charting the LifeCourse framework was explicitly designed to help individuals with IDD and their families develop a vision for their life, and to plan to achieve that vision with the requisite information, skills, and supports they need. The framework's fundamental principles are grounded in the core belief that *all people have the right to live, love, work, play and pursue their life aspirations just as others do in their community.* These principles often influence people to think differently and to inform policy and practice, with the recent promise to broaden the scope of service systems to expand response options to meet people's needs. Since a majority of persons with IDD may not receive formal supports, this framework is broad enough to apply universally to anyone, regardless of whether one has a disability or not. Groups or individuals can use this holistic, person-centered approach to reframe policies and practices within and outside of the disability field, which provides greater versatility for enhancing informal and natural support networks for the person and their family. In addition, the framework supports a focus on practice, policy, and cultural change within organizations and within society to enhance overall quality of life across the life course using the key principles listed below.

3.3.1 Person Within the Context of the Family and Their Community

Although we often view people with IDD as part of their family and community, this has not always been the case, nor is it universally so in the present day due to the many factors that have disrupted this context for people with disabilities and their families. The Charting the LifeCourse principle of a "person within the context of their family and community" can address the needs of each individual member while also recognizing the connections to the family unit, regardless of where the person lives or who they currently have contact with. As a person with IDD defines who they consider their family and describes the reciprocal roles that distinguish their relationships, this highlights that each person in the family unit has their own unique identities, strengths, needs, life cycle, and trajectory that interacts with and contributes to the family dynamic. Although people with disabilities are less likely to be segregated from life within or near their families in the present day, even supports within the community can inadvertently create barriers. Current state and federal disability policies designed to ensure health and safety can have unintended consequences that can prohibit family and community members from maintaining and developing relationships with a person with IDD. For example, the Health Insurance, Portability and Accountability Act (HIPAA) designed to safeguard medical information and private data, can prevent family members from hearing stories from staff about the day-to-day happenings. Friends and co-workers may not know someone's birthday to host a celebration, if the person is receiving disability services, depending on how literal an agency or provider implements HIPAA. Neighbors or other community members are often discouraged from informal interactions because of formal background checks, or state rules and regulations. This contextual principle applies to essential support networks that meet day-to-day needs, but the goal is to integrate supports so that individuals with IDD and families can live interdependently as part of their communities.

3.3.2 Supporting Families' Informational, Socio-Emotional and Day-To-Day Needs

Rather than relying on the delivery of goods and services alone, people with IDD and their families need to actively use targeted supports (e.g. resources and strategies) to get their day-to-day emotional, physical, and material needs met as well as to promote the development, education, interests, and personal well-being of a person and that enhances individual and family functioning. Family members have a key role in the provision of support and guidance to their family member, and as such, supports that benefit the family unit ultimately benefit the individual as well. The Charting the LifeCourse framework addresses supports within three categories; Discovery and Navigation, Connecting and Networking, and Goods and Services (traditionally the formal system of supports). Formal systems of supports have traditionally been less effective to address equally important informational and emotional needs for people and their families (Fairbrother, 2011; Lipman & Longino, 1982).

3.3.3 Holistic Focus Across Interconnected Life Domains

Individuals and families focus on life experiences that point trajectories toward a preferred quality of life. This holistic principle addresses current support structures that focus on self-determination, community living, social capital and economic sufficiency, with an emphasis on planning for life outcomes, not just services. This principle refers to developing a vision for and pursuing a good life, as defined by the person with IDD and their family. It includes providing opportunities to discover what is most important to them, their likes and dislikes, and what they desire for their future. It is rooted in the idea that receiving services and supports is not the outcome, but rather a means to achieve the vision for a good life.

People lead whole lives made up of specific and integrated life domains that are important to a good quality of life, including daily living/employment, safety and security, community living, healthy lifestyle, social and spirituality, and participation and advocacy. The connections across domains are complex and multi-faceted. For example, what happens in one area of life (i.e., job stability) affects another (i.e., housing options). This recognition of the interconnectedness of everyday life helps to broaden the focus across life domains to ensure that individuals with IDD can lead whole lives that are as complete and fulfilling as possible. The life domains described in Table 2 provide a guide to explore the person's strengths, contributions, needs, and wishes across all facets of life and identify pathways to enhance particular domains and achieve a balance. The Charting the Life-Course framework approaches the needs of individuals with disabilities

Table 2 LifeCourse Domains and Definitions

Domain Names	Definition
Daily Life Employment	What a person does as a part of everyday life; school, employment, volunteering, communication, routines, life skills.
Community Living	Where and how someone lives; housing and living options, community access, transportation, home adaptation, and modification.
Social and Spirituality	Building friendships and relationship, leisure activities, personal networks, and faith community.
Healthy Living	Managing and accessing health care and staying well - medical, mental health, behavior, developmental, wellness, and nutrition.
Safety and Security	Staying safe and secure; emergencies, well-being, supported decision-making options, legal rights and issues.
Participation and Advocacy	Participating in community life and having a valued role - self-advocacy, voting and contribution.

and their families through multiple life domains, rather than a single, narrow life domain. Exploring all possibilities within this listing of life domains will ensure that one person's focus does not narrow to any one area such as health and safety at the expense of limiting exploration of a broad array of domains that ensure a good life. Individuals with disabilities and their families are continually juggling a number of variables to enhance their quality of life (Hewitt, Agosta, Williams, & Reinke, 2013).

3.3.4 Trajectory for Enhancing Life Experiences

The concept for the Life Stage Trajectory principle is built on the concept that people move through a series of life stages beginning with infancy and then on through early childhood, school age, transition age, adulthood, and older adulthood. Each stage encompasses growth and experiential learning that builds over time to impact the next stage. Individuals and families can focus on a specific life stage with an awareness of how experiences in that stage influence what happens in the future. Another part of this principle focuses on creating a trajectory toward a good life as defined by the person with IDD and their family. Plotting this course, helps to ensure that necessary building blocks are in place for each stage. For example, if a person has a goal of working in the community, early learning experiences that can contribute to their success such as being responsible for household chores and navigating relationships with peers. With anticipatory guidance, families can proactively consider the types of activities and experiences that will help forge the path toward a positive trajectory.

Regarding this LifeCourse principle, people with IDD may not experience equal opportunities to have experiences or make mistakes across life stages that lead to practical learning and development. Risk taking can be about internal or external elements in one's life (Robertson & Collison, 2011). For example, a person with IDD may not have the opportunity to try a new position at work because an employer may think that they cannot perform the duties of this job without harm. At other times, a family may not let their son or daughter take the local bus to their grandparent's home since they might make a mistake and get off at the wrong stop. Embedded in this principle is an awareness of the necessity of these opportunities for people with IDD to learn and grow from their experiences and to make mistakes just as others do. These experiences serve a purpose and contribute to a full and meaningful life.

Initially, people with IDD may need help to construct a vision for a good life.

Generating ideas to construct this vision may not be readily available to people with IDD. One way to start this conversation could be to ask what someone *does not want* — a much easier question to answer. The individual may be able to clearly state that they do not want to live in a segregated living setting, but may need assistance exploring alternatives available to them. As is commonplace for any family, the parent's ideal trajectory and individual's ideal trajectory might be considerably different and may require adjustment over time.

3.3.5 Integrating Services and Supports Across the Life Span

A key component of Charting the LifeCourse framework is the Integrated Supports Star, a tool to help people and their families visualize and combine different kinds of supports as options to include in plotting their trajectory toward an inclusive, high quality life in the place where they live or community of their choice. In order to support a good life, a person with IDD can draw from (a) Personal Strengths and Assets (things owned, skills learned, personal qualities); (b) Relationships (family, friends, community connections); (c) Eligibility Specific supports (disability or needs-based supports, if available); (d) Community Based supports (places, groups, public resources); and/or (e) Technology supports. Personal technology can be mainstream or specialized assistive devices; environmental technology — smart homes, transportation, bionics, and/or assistive technology — screen readers, visual prompts, adaptive equipment or hearing aids. This strategy allows for day-to-day problem solving or planning for services now and in the future.

Individuals and families utilize an array of integrated supports to achieve the envisioned good life, including the individual's strengths and assets, relationship based supports, technology, and community supports. In addition, people with IDD may have public or privately funded supports based on eligibility. The basis of this principle encourages people with IDD, their families, and those who support them to first identify the support need, and then consider the most effective source of support to achieve the desired life outcome. We describe each of the five primary sources of support included in this principle below (Fig. 1).

Consider a person identifying supports to meet transportation needs. Oftentimes, the options include family members, disability-specific options, and public transportation, if available. Using the five support components of the star, one would explore each option individually and then strategize to integrate or leverage the options to meet all of the transportation needs of

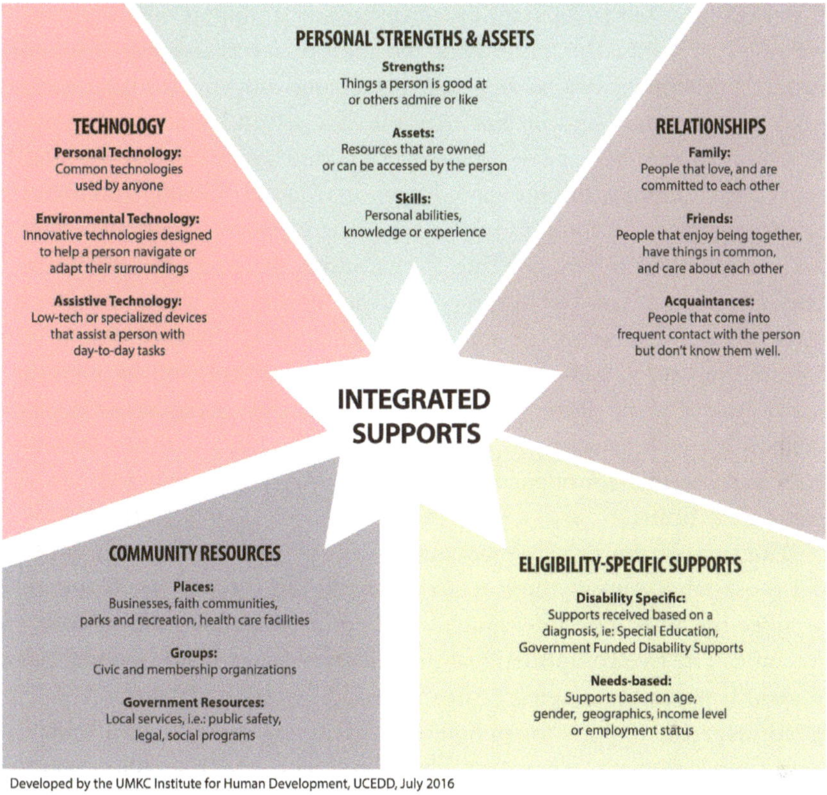

Figure 1 Charting the lifecourse integrated services and supports star

the person. For example, is the person able to navigate different forms of transportation or to build their capacity for doing this on their own? Are there people that assist with driving a person to and from where they need to go or to set up a carpool? Is there accessible public transit or are communities walkable or bike-friendly? Technology can involve use of transportation apps (Uber/Lyft) or virtual mobility aids for using public transit. What government programs or services are available to fund or fill the transportation gap?

When considering supports for a person with 24-hour needs, families often believe the only options are residential supports or no formal supports at all. The Charting the LifeCourse framework and tools can be used to problem-solve and plan with persons with IDD and their families to identify outcomes that lead to their good life, as they define it, and then using the Integrated Supports Star to navigate the services and supports to achieve it. Person-centered facilitators, case-managers and support coordinators are learning how to use the framework and tools to access an array of supports for each outcome area, as opposed to relying only on formal disability supports as the only option. For example, if a person has access to funding for a limited number of self-directed hours but has needs that require 24 hours a day supports, the Integrated Supports Star can identify and leverage other supports to fill the gaps beyond the paid supports. Using the different components of the star, one family that assists their son in self-directing services color-codes a weekly calendar that coordinates whether paid supports, technology, family, or community supports are in place during each hour of the day. In addition, the family emphasizes the need to build their son's capacity to be alone for short periods by increasing use of personal technology, such as iPad and telephone with the hope that this builds his skills, and parental confidence, for using remote monitoring or other supports in the future.

The basis of this principle encourages people with IDD, their families, and those who support them to first identify the support need, and then consider the most effective source of support to achieve the desired life outcome. The five components of the integrated star provide a visual guide to identifying and leveraging across options for every hour of the day. This broad range of supports for people with IDD and their families shifts the focus from complete reliance on eligibility-based or relationship-based to viewing them as options among a larger network of supports available. Another significant contribution related to this principle is an exploration of sources of support that begins with the person and their abilities, strengths, and assets. Focusing first on the person's strengths, talents, and interests maintains a person-centered, individualized approach to supports as well as promotes independence and choice.

4. REFRAMING CHANGE TO FOCUS ON INTEGRATED SUPPORTS

If we aspire to fulfill the Position Statement on Community Living and Participation (AAIDD & AUCD, 2016) that "Everyone with [IDD] deserves to live in the community where they have the opportunity to experience vibrant lives that include work, friends, family, and high expectations for community contributions", there is work to do. Charting the LifeCourse framework provides a means to address integrated supports and infuse self-determined principles of choice, decision-making, problem solving, and goal setting into a person-centered trajectory. Using a number of areas on the Integrated Supports Star can affect quality of life for the person and family, influence formal supports through policy and legislation, and improve aspects of living in the community.

Family networks are incorporating the framework and accompanying tools into training workshops that enhance family skills and knowledge to navigate integrated supports for all its members. Families utilize the tools to capture their hopes, dreams, and fears for their child while discovering what is possible for the future. A local organization in rural Northwest Missouri connects families with a Family Navigator who uses the framework and tools when meeting one-to-one with families to learn how to use the Integrated Supports Star principle to connect and leverage their own resources with informal supports (technology, community, and people in their lives) and formal disability-specific supports. A father worked to connect successfully to local recreational supports for his child with Autism to help with after school care while learning about the formal supports he can access when needed. In Pennsylvania, Family Leaders are educating groups of families on the quality of life principle that focuses on possibilities for the future and building their capacity to create opportunities for life experiences that will enhance friendships, social capital and self-determination not only for their current situation but also for the future. In South Dakota, families are using the framework to learn to advocate for their children in formal planning meetings by utilizing the trajectory principle that focuses on creating a vision for a good life while reflecting on past positive and negative life experiences and begins to define the current goals. The principles are providing a common language for communicating what they believe is important to, and for their child with a disability. Families are also learning how to help their child express his/her own hopes, dreams, and fears and how those may be different from their own.

Formal disability support programs used the Charting the LifeCourse framework to consider the entire population of people with IDD to enhance the current policy and systems change initiatives. The framework provides stakeholders foundational language and understanding of key concepts within disability field that have been otherwise hard to understand. For example, an infographic was developed to illustrate the fact that the majority of people with IDD do not receive formal paid services from the state agency and is being used for strategic planning that focuses on changes within the state system but also the need to partner and leverage partnerships outside of the DD system. This is important because it reframes how the system understands and responds to people with IDD and their families that are not currently receiving supports. It is important to recognize (a) some number of these individuals may request IDD services in the future, (b) members of this group may be utilizing effective strategies and resources within their communities that keep them from turning to formal services, and (c) that formal systems for support may not offer what individuals and families need.

Individuals with IDD and their families have experience and knowledge of the strengths and barriers of integrating supports to meet their needs. By including families in determining individual support needs, as well as systems change efforts, we can honor the experiences of families and people with disabilities and capture their concerns, needs, strengths, and ideas to integrate supports. The framework provides a shared vision and language for bringing together self-advocates, families and professionals around a common purpose and co-create solutions. For systems change, CoP teams used the framework and tools to design opportunities to share their stories, participate and lead family focus groups and meetings, and develop side-by-side training workshops with professionals that provided a platform for developing policy and practice changes in their state. Several states established or reinvigorated self-advocate and family advisory councils for their state agencies. Successful models of inclusion included provisions to accommodate their participation such as stipends, child-care, or convenient community locations.

CoP Teams applied the Charting the LifeCourse Framework to transform the long-term service systems to enhance supports to persons with IDD and their families. For example, the Tennessee CoP team uses the framework to guide the development of a new waiver to serve more people and promote employment and community inclusion by leveraging informal supports with self-directed supports offered in the Home and Community Based (HCBS) waiver that would fill in gaps of need. Additionally, Peer-to-Peer Support and Family-to-Family Support provided a structure to connect people with IDD and families with peers who have had successful experiences with employment. Peer-to-peer support is a way to connect with others who are experiencing the same problems. Family-to-Family Support is essentially support from peers that are part of a family. This informal connection with others who are feeling stress or social isolation tends to improve social relationships and provides emotional support (Bray, Carter, Sanders, Blake, & Keegan, 2017). The integrated support star principle serves as the foundation for understanding how self-directed supports offered in the HCBS waiver may combine with informal supports to meet the support needs. Funding for families to access family-to-family support and family training designed to provide a structure to connect people with IDD and families with peers who have had successful experiences with employment and accessing integrated supports is also included in the Tennessee waiver. Likewise, in Oklahoma, the framework guided the CoP team in the development of recommendations for the Governor's Blue Ribbon Panel on the Waiting List. Each guiding principle reframed the panels' understanding of those on the waiting list and possible solutions they had not considered before. Utilizing the integrated star, the panel recommendations focused on not only disability specific government programs, but also enhancing access to other social service government programs that did not traditionally provide supports to people with disabilities. Understanding that families have needs beyond only goods and services, a new initiatives centered around the information and navigation needs of persons with IDD and their families throughout the lifespan in accessing both paid or eligibility-specific supports and unpaid supports. The District of Columbia CoP also recognized the utility of the framework for transforming the long-term service and support system and introduced concepts and tools as part of the District's "No Wrong Door" initiative for application universally across departments and populations with long-term support needs. Front Door staff and Options Counselors train on the framework and tools utilizing the integrated support star categories to reframe and organize the conversations with families in need of supports. This not only identifies current family supports but also maps ideas for building options within paid and unpaid services.

The Charting the LifeCourse framework, which provides a holistic, life span approach that is universal to any target population, provides a platform for stakeholders to realize and form new alliances and work together on common goals that reach beyond disability. Through communication strategies and other efforts, many CoP sites were able to attract new partners beyond disability specific partners. For example, the District of Columbia team formed a partnership with Georgetown University and a local law firm to address common goals to implement supported decision-making, as an alternative to guardianship. Focusing on the people in a person's life that know them best, and identifying strategies for enhancing these relationships is at the center of supported decision making. The Oklahoma team collaborated with the state's largest school district to offer resources based on the framework to educators. Educators were less aware of the supports for transitioning youth beyond traditional adult formal supports. By providing education and training on how to apply the framework to outcomes identified during the IEP process, students had plans that integrated supports beyond disability-specific supports. The Tennessee team formed working relationships with managed care organizations charged with managing a new waiver to serve individuals with IDD living in their own home or family home. Support coordinators developed plans that leveraged family resources with community and formal supports. Additionally, an organization in Missouri invested in family support by worked closely with community partners to build an inclusive playground in the middle of town. The hope is that providing an inclusive environment for children to run and play alongside their peers while parents are connecting to other parents will increase the natural supports and friendships.

5. CURRENT STATUS AND FUTURE DIRECTIONS FOR THE INTEGRATED SUPPORTS PARADIGM

The promise of integrated supports for people IDD is becoming reality in the many applications of the Charting the LifeCourse framework. The initial use and expansion of the CoP on Charting the LifeCourse principles and practices engaged stakeholders at all levels: person, family, community, research, and policy. This framework promotes a good life for people and their families while offering a way to organize and arrive at innovative, values-driven solutions to common issues that families experience at any life stage. In addition, the principles of the LifeCourse framework resonate with a broad audience to establish new partnerships with common goals supporting people and families (Reynolds & Kardell, 2017). In addition, the framework's common language unites stakeholders across disciplines and age ranges to organize and implement strategies that permit scaling up activities beyond the immediate scope of CoP participation. The paradigm shift represented by the CoP may be a pivotal moment in the field of IDD (Reynolds & Kardell, 2017). New alliances and collective efforts to support people with IDD and their families encourages a reconceptualization of integrated supports as described below.

6. CONCLUSION

Thompson, Schalock, Agosta, Teninty, and Fortune (2014) wrote that one of the "inconvenient realities" is that finite resources, rather than enough money limit funding mechanisms for people with IDD for all.

At all ages and stages of life, public funding is generally inadequate to serve all who qualify. Rather than broadly share available funds, the primary solution is for some people to get some level of formal supports while others get none. Using natural supports in combination with or without formal funding for people with IDD can still work toward achieving a good life with help from friends, family, professionals, community members, and people we meet over time by using natural supports in the activities within environments that they choose.

Although providing natural supports is viewed as a task for long-time friends and relatives or a place to go in the community, Boissenvain (1968) challenged social scientists to consider a broader system of social interaction nuanced through coalitions of persons in less-formalized groups. For example, people may not know everyone in a network or interest group, or a particular segment of the community, but this vague and unstable social form is an important aspect of living in the community and people with IDD can benefit from this type of informal support. Boissenvain argues that these less stable collections of persons are less observable than typical groups with long-term social relations, but these informal networks that people move within and around are also capable of providing natural supports.

Aspects to initiate and sustain efforts to realign systems of support include catalysts to prompt change, and underlying system infrastructure and drivers to institute exemplary approaches. Within the metaphor of stable paid or eligibility-specific supports, natural supports seem less stable, less important, or even too unpredictable to ensure health and safety in contrast with formal supports. However, if we deepen our understanding of what we mean by "natural supports", and truly focus on intentionally helping persons with IDD and their families to develop and sustain integrated support structures, our field we will move closer to fully actualizing a formal person-centered services and supports system. This system should align with Article 1 of the UN Convention on the Rights of People with Disabilities to *promote, protect and ensure the full and equal enjoyment of all human rights and fundamental freedoms by all persons with disabilities, and to promote respect for their inherent dignity*.

To achieve this, we must stop perpetuating the myth or misaligned social contract that formal eligibility-specific paid supports are the only means to achieving a desired quality of life for persons with disabilities and begin to help people utilize formal long-term services and supports as a way of enhancing, leveraging, or connecting around the person's system of informal supports. Approaches to support must adapt to the ever-evolving life cycle of the family and life stage of individual members. To effectively use formal supports to enhance natural or informal supports involves (a) recognizing and enhancing a person's capacities, (b) strengthening and connecting social networks, (c) leveraging resources within environments accessed by all citizens, (d) utilizing technological innovations so people with IDD can achieve their preferred quality of life. Wehmeyer and Shogren (2017) concur that technology is critically important in building skills for community living and social interaction.

Historically, sources of support people with IDD were either natural support or formal, eligibility-specific paid services. The concept of natural supports was often synonymous with unpaid supports or support by family members as part of their role. However, an international literature review on natural supports (National Disability Authority, 2011) yielded little information until adding the search term, social networks/social support, to indicate the need for others to support employment, daily living skills, and community participation. Early literature on natural supports (1970s) focused on family and friends of a person with IDD to support independent living, but most recently natural supports are referred to in supported employment (Butterworth et al., 2016). Employment is just one example of an area in which there must be a flexible plan for services and supports to meet the needs of people in the current and future workforce, since there is less stability or predictability related to occupations and individual progressions within a single industry or particular company. Traditional practices within career counseling and vocational support must now adapt to the complexity of human life and meet diversity of the workforce and the need for jobs in the community (Wehmeyer et al., 2018). Nota and Soresi (2012) identified that higher levels of adaptability within people with and without disabilities tended to predict a positive attitude toward the future that could involve making changes in initial plans, personal improvement, and learning additional skills and knowledge.

In conclusion, to best support people with disabilities and their families, natural supports should be a logical and efficient integration of available supports, as opposed to a dichotomy of only two options - paid and natural. Natural supports are linkages of the following: 1) *Personal Capacity* of the person with disabilities, 2) *Relationship-Based Social Networks,* 3) *Environmental Structures*, and 4) *Technology-Enhanced supports and when combined with Eligibility-Specific supports, if available to create a good life.* The cycle of planning and implementation of trajectories within the LifeCourse provide a means to effectively direct and integrate self-selected natural supports and the limited amount of paid eligibility-specific services, if available to be able to live, laugh, love, and work in a community of their choice, within their family circle.

ACKNOWLEDGMENTS

The Community of Practice for Supporting Families of Individuals with Intellectual & Developmental Disabilities is a national initiative of the University of Missouri Kansas City-Institute on Human Development, University Center in Developmental Disabilities and the National Association of State Directors of Developmental Disabilities Services. This project was funded in part by the Administration on Intellectual and Developmental Disabilities grant 90DN0298 and the effort is now sustained through a statewide membership structure. Grantees undertaking projects under government sponsorship and their evaluators are encouraged to express freely their findings and conclusions. Points of view or opinions do not, therefore, necessarily represent official positions of the University of Missouri-Kansas City, or any partners or funding sources. The authors wish to thank Yoshi Kardell of Human Services Research Institute, Jane St. John, Katherine Ragon, and Rachel Hiles of UMKC for their contributions to the article. We are grateful for their work on the Charting the LifeCourse initiatives.

REFERENCES

AAIDD, & AUCD. (2016). *Community living and participation for people with intellectual and developmental disabilities.* Retrieved from: http://aaidd.org/news-policy/policy/position-statements/community-living-and-participation#.Wr08hJch1PY.

Amado, A. N., Stancliffe, R. J., McCarron, M., & McCallion, P. (2013). Social inclusion and community participation of individuals with intellectual/developmental disabilities. *Intellectual and Developmental Disabilities, 51*, 360–375.

Bailey, L., & Nixon, Y. M. (2014). Support planning success stories from a provider organization's journey. *Inclusion, 2*, 110–124. https://doi.org/10.1352/2326-6988-2.2.110.

Boissenvain, J. (1968). The place of non-groups in the social sciences. In *Man, new series* (Vol. 3, pp. 542–556). London: Royal Anthropological Institutes of Great Britain and Ireland. Retrieved from: http://www.jstor.org/stable/2798578.

Bowen, M., & Kerr, M. (1988). *Family evaluation.* New York: W.W. Norton & Company.

Bray, L., Carter, B., Sanders, C., Blake, L., & Keegan. (2017). Parent-to-parent peer support for parents of children with a disability: A mixed method study. *Patient Education and Counseling, 100*, 1537–1543. https://doi.org/10.1016/j.ped.2017.03.004.

Bronfenbrenner, U. (1989). Ecological systems theory. In R. Vasta (Ed.), *Annals of child development* (Vol. 6, pp. 187–224). Greenwich, CT: JAI.

Brown, I., Radford, J. P., & Wehmeyer, M. L. (2017a). Historical overview of intellectual and developmental disabilities. In M. L. Wehmeyer, I. Borwn, M. Percy, K. A. Shogren, & W. L. A. Fung (Eds.), *A comprehensive guide to intellectual and developmental disabilities* (pp. 19–34). Baltimore, MD: Brookes Publishing.

Brown, I., Wehmeyer, M. L., & Shogren, K. A. (2017b). What is meant by the terms intellectual disability and developmental disabilities? In M. L. Wehmeyer, I. Borwn, M. Percy, K. A. Shogren, & W. L. A. Fung (Eds.), *A comprehensive guide to intellectual and developmental disabilities* (pp. 3–18). Baltimore, MD: Brookes Publishing.

Buntinx, W. H. E. (2013). Understanding disability: A strengths-based approach. In M. L. Wehmeyer (Ed.), *The Oxford handbook of positive psychology and disability* (pp. 7–18). New York: Oxford University Press.

Buntinx, W. H. E., & Schalock, R. L. (2010). Models of disability, quality of life, and individualized supports: Implications for professional practice in intellectual disability. *Journal of Policy and Practice in Intellectual Disabilities, 7*, 283–294.

Butterworth, J., Smith, F. A., Winsor, J., Ciulla Timmons, J., Migliore, A., & Domin, D. (2016). *State Data: The national report on employment services and outcomes.* Boston, MA: University of Massachusetts Boston, Institute for Community Inclusion.

Charting the LifeCourse framework.(2017). Retrieved from: http://www.lifecoursetools.com/principles/.

Claes, C., Van Hove, G., Vandevelde, S., van Loon, J., & Schalock, R. L. (2010). Person-centered planning: Analysis of research and effectiveness. *Intellectual and Developmental Disabilities, 48*, 432–453. https://doi.org/10.1352/1934-9556-48.6.432.

Developmental Disabilities Assistance and Bill of Rights Act Amendments of 2000, PL 106-402, 42 U.S.C. §§ 6000 et seq.

Dinerstein, R. D. (2012). Implementing legal capacity under Article 12 of the UN convention on the rights of persons with Disabilities: The difficult road from guardianship to supported decision-making. *Human Rights Brief, 19*(2), 9.

Dinerstein, R. D. (2016). The Olmstead imperative: The right to live in the community and beyond. *Inclusion, 4*, 16–20. https://doi.org/10.1352/2326-6988-4.1.16.

Duggan, C., & Linehan, C. (2013). The role of 'natural supports' in promoting independent living for people with disabilities: A review of existing literature. *British Journal of Learning Disabilities, 414*, 199–207.

Duncan, M. K. W., & Blugis, A. (2011). Maslow's needs hierarchy as a framework for evaluating hospitality houses' resources and services. *Journal of Pediatric Nursing, 26*, 325–331.

Dunst, C. J., & Bruder, M. B. (2002). Valued outcomes of service coordination, early intervention, and natural environments. *Exceptional Children, 68*, 361–375.

Elder, G. H. (1998). The life course as developmental theory. *Child Development, 69*, 1–12.

Elder, G. H., Johnson, M. K., & Crosnoe, R. (2003). The emergence and development of life course theory. In J. T. Mortimer, & M. J. Shanaham (Eds.), *Handbook of the life course* (pp. 3–19). New York: Plenum.

Fairbrother, N. (2011). Social support. *Visions, 6*(4), 7–10. Retrieved from: https://www.heretohelp.bc.ca/sites/default/files/images/visions-ss.pdf.

Ferguson, D. L., Ferguson, P. M., & Wehmeyer, M. L. (2013). The self-advocacy movement. In M. L. Wehmeyer (Ed.), *The story of intellectual disability* (pp. 233–277). Baltimore, MD: Brookes Publishing.

Friedman, C., & Spassiani, N. A. (2017). Getting out there: Community support services for people with intellectual and developmental disabilities in Medicaid HCBS waivers. *Inclusion, 5*, 33–44.

Gotto, G. S., Calkins, C. F., Jackson, L., Walker, H., & Beckman, C. (2010). *Accessing social Capital: Implications for persons with disabilities.* Retrieved from: http://www.aucd.org/NGSD/template/link.cfm.

Hecht, E., Reynolds, M., Agosta, J., & McGinley, K. (2011). *Building an agenda for supporting families with a member with intellectual and developmental disabilities. Report of the Wingspread Conference on building a family support agenda, March 6-8, 2011.* Racine, Wisconsin: Johnson Foundation.

Hewitt, A. (2014). Presidential address, 2014-embracing Complexity: Community inclusion, participation and citizenship. *Intellectual and Developmental Disabilities, 52*, 475–495. https://doi.org/10.1352/1934-9556-52.6.475.

Hewitt, A., Agosta, J., Williams, A. C., & Reinke, J. (2013). Families of individuals with intellectual and developmental disabilities: Policy funding, services, and experiences. *Intellectual and Developmental Disabilities, 51*, 349–359. https://doi.org/10.1352/1934-9556-51.5.349.

Hurst, K. F., Ramsdell, C. P., & Sorice, M. G. (2017). A lifecourse approach to understanding social drivers of rangeland conversion. *Ecology and Society, 22*. Retrieved from: https://doi.org/10.5751/ES-08990-220119.

Hutchinson, E. D. (2015). Human behavior: A multidimensional approach. In E. D. Huchinson (Ed.), *Dimensions of human behavior: Person and environment* (5th ed., pp. 1–38). Thousand Oaks, CA: Sage.

Jameson, J. M., Riesen, T., Polychronis, S., Trader, B., Mizner, S., Martinis, J., & Hoyle, D. (2015). Guardianship and the potential of supported decision making with individuals with disabilities. *Research and Practice for Persons with Severe Disabilities*, 1–16. https://doi.org/10.1177/1540796915586189.

Klein, J., & Strully, J. L. (2000). From unit d to the community: A dream to fulfill. In M. L. Wehmeyer, & J. R. Patton (Eds.), *Mental retardation in the 21st century* (pp. 165–178). Austin, TX: Pro-Ed.

Lachapelle, Y., Wehmeyer, M. L., Haelewyck, M. C., Courbois, Y., Keith, K. D., Schalock, & Walsh, P. N. (2005). The relationship between quality of life and self-determination: An international study. *Journal of Intellectual Disability Research: JIDR, 49*, 740–744.

Larson, S. A., Eschenbacher, H. J., Anderson, L. L., Taylor, B., Pettingell, S., Hewitt, A., ... Bourne, M. L. (November 2017). *In-home and residential long-term supports and services for persons with intellectual or developmental disabilities: Status and trends through 2015*. Minneapolis: University of Minnesota, Research and Training Center on Community Living, Institute on Community Integration. Retrieved from: http://nasuad.org/sites/nasuad/files/2015_RISP-WEB.pdf.

Lipman, A., & Longino, C. F. (1982). Formal and informal support: A conceptual clarification. *Journal of Applied Gerontology, 1*, 141–146.

Luckasson, R., Borthwick-Duffy, S., Buntinx, W. H. E., Coulter, D. L., Croiag, E., & Reeve, A. (2002). *Mental retardation: Definition, classification, and systems of support* (10th ed.). Washington, DC: AAMR.

Martin, L., Grandia, P., Ouellette-Kuntz, H., & Cobigo, V. (2016). From framework to practice: Person-directed planning in the real world. *Journal of Applied Research in Intellectual Disabilities, 29*, 552–565. https://doi.org/10.1111/jar.12214.

Maslow, A. (1970). *Motivation and personality* (2nd ed.). New York: Harper and Row.

National Alliance for Caregiving, & AARP Public Policy Institute. (2015). *Research Report: Caregiving in the US*. Retrieved from: http:ww1.prweb.com/prfiles/2015/06/03/12765231/2015_Caqregivinginthe_US_Final%20Report_WEB.pdf.

National Disability Authority. (September 2011). *A review of literature on natural community supports: A contemporary developments in disability services paper*. Retrieved from: http://nda.ie/nda-files/A-Review-of-Literature-on-Natural-Community-Supports1.pdf.

Noll, S., Smith, D. J., & Wehmeyer, M. L. (2013). In search of science: Intellectual disability in late modern times. In M. L. Wehmeyer (Ed.), *The story of intellectual disability* (pp. 117–156). Baltimore, MD: Brookes Publishing.

Noltemeyer, A., Bush, K., Patton, J. M., & Bergen, D. (2012). The relationship among deficiency needs and growth needs: An empirical investigation of Maslow's theory. *Children and Youth Services Review, 34*, 1862–7867. https://doi.org/10.1016/j.childyouth.2012.05.021.

Nota, L., & Soresi, S. (September 2012). *Career adaptability, hope and optimism in adults with and without disability. Paper presented at the Life Design and Career Counseling Seminars*. Padova, Italy: University of Padova.

O'Brien, J., & Pearpoint, J. (2002). *Person-centered planning with MAPS and PATH. A workbook for facilitators*. Toronto: Inclusion Press.

Palmer, S. B. (2010). Self-Determination – a life-span perspective. *Focus on Exceptional Children, 42*, 1–16.

Palmer, S. B., & Turnbull, H. R. (October 2012). A blueprint for building social capital. In S. Palmer, T. Heller, G. Gotto, J. Peterson-Besse, & S. Reynolds (Eds.), *Research to practice in self-determination: Family focus on self-determination* (pp. 24–26). Retrieved from: http://ngsd.org/sites/default/files/research_to_practice_sd_-_issue_4.pdf.

Park, J., Marquis, J., Hoffman, L., TurnbuU, A., Poston, D., … Nelson, L. (2003). Assessing family quality of life as the service outcome. *Journal of Intellectual Disability Research: JIDR, 47*(5), 367–384.

Poston, D. J., Turnbull, A. P., Park, J., Mannan, H., Marquis, J., & Wang, M. (2003). Family quality of life: A qualitative inquiry. *Mental Retardation, 41*, 313–328. https://doi.org/10.1352/0047-6765(2003)414-313.

Reynolds, M. C. (December 2015). *Issue Brief: Supporting families of people with IDD*. Washington, DC: AAIDD. Retrieved from: http://aaidd.org/docs/default-source/National-Goals/supporting-families-of-people-with-idd.pdf?sfvrsn=0.

Reynolds, M. C., Gotto, G. S., Arnold, C., Boehm, T. L., Magana, S., Dinora, P., … Shaffert, R. (2015). National goals for supporting families across the life course. *Inclusion, 3*, 260–266. https://doi.org/10.1352/2326-6988-3.4.260.

Reynolds, M. C., & Kardell, Y. (2017). Charting the LifeCourse for persons with IDD and their families: Moving from principles to practice. *Social Innovations Journal, 32*, 20–33.

Reynolds, M. C., St John, J., & Gotto, G. (October 2012). Scaling up self-determination through family support. In S. Palmer, T. Heller, G. Gotto, J. Peterson-Besse, & S. Reynolds (Eds.), *Research to practice in self-determination: Family focus on self-determination* (pp. 24–26). Retrieved from: http://ngsd.org/sites/default/files/research_to_practice_sd_-_issue_4.pdf.

Rich, A. J. (2015). *Standing together and finding a voice apart: Advocating for intellectual disability rights*. Washington, DC: AAIDD.

Robertson, J. P., & Collison, C. (2011). Positive risk taking: Whose risk is it? An exploration in community outreach teams in adult mental health and learning disability services. *Health, Risk & Society, 13*, 147–164.

Rothbaum, F., Rosen, K., Ujiie, T., & Uchida, N. (2002). Family systems theory, attachment theory, and culture. *Family Process, 41*, 328–350.

Schalock, R. L. (2000). Three decades of quality of life. In M. L.Wehmeyer, & J. R. Patton (Eds.), *Mental retardation in the 21st century* (pp. 335–358). Austin, TX: ProEd.

Schalock, R. L., Borthwick-Duffey, S., Bradley, V., Buntinx, W., Coulter, D., Craig, E., … Wehmeyer, M. (2010). *Intellectual disability: Definition, classification, and systems of supports* (11th ed.). Washington, DC: American Association on Intellectual and Developmental Disabilities.

Shogren, K. A., Wehmeyer, M. L., Palmer, S. B., Forber-Pratt, A. J., Little, T. J., & Lopez, S. (2015). Causal agency theory: Reconceptualizing a functional model of self-determination. *Education and Training in Autism and Developmental Disabilities, 50*, 251–263.

Smith, J. D., & Wehmeyer, M. L. (2012). *Good blood, bad blood: Science, nature and the myth of the Kallikaks*. Washington, DC: AAIDD.

Summers, J. A., Hoffman, L., Marquis, J., Turnbull, A., Poston, D., & Nelson, L. L. (2005). Measuring the quality of family-professional partnerships in special education services. *Exceptional Children, 72*, 65–81.

Thompson, J. R., Bradley, V. J., Buntinx, W. H. E., Schalock, R. L., Shogren, K. A., Snell, M. E., … Yeager, M. H. (2009). Conceptualizing supports and the support needs of people with intellectual disability. *Intellectual and Developmental Disabilities, 47*, 135–146. https://doi.org/10.1352/1934-9556-47.2135.

Thompson, J. R., Schalock, R. L., Agosta, J., Teninty, L., & Fortune, J. (2014). How the supports paradigm is transforming the developmental disabilities service system. *Inclusion, 2*, 86–99. https://doi.org/10.1352/2326-6988-2.2.86.

Tichá, R., Hewitt, A., Nord, D., & Larson, S. (2013). System and individual outcomes and their predictors in services and support for people with IDD. *Intellectual and Developmental Disabilities, 51*, 298–315.

Turnbull, A., Brown, I., & Turnbull, H. R. (2004). *Families and people with mental retardation and quality of life: International perspectives*. Washington, DC: American Association on Mental Retardation.

Turnbull, H. R., & Turnbull, A. P. (2000). Family support: Retrospective and prospective. In M. L. Wehmeyer, & J. R. Patton (Eds.), *Mental retardation in the 21st century* (pp. 3–17). Austin, TX: ProEd.

Turnbull, A., Turnbull, H. R., Erwin, E. J., Soodak, L. C., & Shogren, K. A. (2015). *Families, professionals, and exceptionality* (7th ed.). Boston: Pearson.

Vandercook, T., York, J., & Froest, M. (1989). The McGill action planning system (MAPS): A strategy for building the vision. *The Journal of the Association for Persons with Severe Handicaps, 14*, 205–215.

Wehmeyer, M. L. (1999). A functional model of self-determination: Describing development and implementing instruction. *Focus on Autism and Other Developmental Disabilities, 14*, 53–61.

Wehmeyer, M. L. (2013). Beyond pathology: Positive psychology and disability. In M. L. Wehmeyer (Ed.), *The Oxford handbook of positive psychology and disability* (pp. 3–6). New York: Oxford University Press.

Wehmeyer, M. L., Agran, M., Hughes, C., Martin, J., Mithaug, D. E., & Palmer, S. (2007). *Promoting self-determination in students with intellectual and developmental disabilities*. New York: Guilford Press.

Wehmeyer, M. L., Bersani, H., & Gagne, R. (2000). Riding the third wave: Self-determination and self-advocacy in the 21st century. In M. L. Wehmeyer, & J. R. Patton (Eds.), *Mental retardation in the 21st century* (pp. 315–333). Austin, TX: PRO-ED.

Wehmeyer, M. L., Nota, L., Soresi, S., Shogren, K. A., Morningstar, M. E., Ferrari, L., … DiMaggio, I. (2018). A crisis in career development: Life designing and implications for transition. *Career Development and Transition for Exceptional Individuals*, 1–9. https://doi.org/10.1177/2165143417750092.

Wehmeyer, M. L., & Schalock, R. L. (2013). The parent movement. In M. L. Wehmeyer (Ed.), *The story of intellectual disability* (pp. 187–231). Baltimore, MD: Brookes Publishing.

Wehmeyer, M. L., & Schwartz, M. (1998). The relationship between self-determination, quality of life, and life satisfaction for adults with mental retardation. *Education and Training in Mental Retardation and Developmental Disabilities, 33*, 3–12.

Wehmeyer, M. L., & Shogren, K. A. (2017). Future trends and advances in intellectual and developmental disabilities. In M. L. Wehmeyer, I. Borwn, M. Percy, K. A. Shogren, & W. L. A. Fung (Eds.), *A comprehensive guide to intellectual and developmental disabilities* (pp. 737–743). Baltimore, MD: Brookes Publishing.

Zalenski, R. J., & Raspa, R. (2006). Maslow's hierarchy of needs: A framework for achieving human potential in hospice. *Journal of Palliative Medicine, 9*, 1120–1127.

CHAPTER SEVEN

Information and Referral Services in IDD: Toward Integrated and Comprehensive Services?

Robert M. Hodapp*[,§,1], Jan Rosemergy*, Bridgette L. Garcia*[,§], Sophie A. Meskis*[,§], Megan Hart* and Elise McMillan*
*Vanderbilt Kennedy Center UCEDD, Nashville, TN, United States
[§]Department of Special Education, Peabody College, Vanderbilt University, Nashville, TN, United States
[1]Corresponding Author: E-mail: robert.hodapp@vanderbilt.edu

Contents

Abstract

Faced with the difficulties that most everyone has in accessing needed social services, information and referral (I&R) services have arisen and gained prominence across the United States. This need for I&R services would seem even more pronounced when dealing with disability services, as disability service-systems are notoriously complex and hard to navigate, with families and individuals experiencing difficulties in learning

International Review of Research in Developmental Disabilities, Volume 54
ISSN 2211-6095
https://doi.org/10.1016/bs.irrdd.2018.07.007

about, becoming eligible for, applying for, and receiving disability services. In this review, we first describe the numerous disability-related services available in education, health, law, employment, adult services, and family support, before examining the nation's I&R movement and how I&R services operate. We then detail one disability-related I&R service, Tennessee Disability Pathfinder, before exploring the future promise and challenges facing such disability-related I&R services. Although woefully under-developed, disability-related I&R services would seem a critical, almost necessary service for parents, individuals, and agencies as they navigate our country's complex and changing disability service systems.

Although opinions differ about modern technologies, most would agree that the World Wide Web has fostered an information revolution. Connecting to the internet via computers, phones, and ipads, users can easily learn about a variety of topics. And yet, while quickly producing web-sites, links, PDF's, and podcasts related to a specific topic, the web has also been criticized for its lack of rules and standards, as well as its propensity toward information over-load (Martland & Rothbaum, 2006). The user has few guidelines as to how to evaluate any of the information produced and the paid links, while they appear at the top of most search-lists, may not necessarily provide helpful or reliable information.

The web's strengths and weaknesses are amply demonstrated with regard to disability services. The strength is that, compared to pre-internet days, the user has access to hundreds or even thousands of potential services. But as has often been noted (Holl & Meyer, 2014; Nageswaran, Parish, Rose, & Grady, 2011), disability services are notoriously hard to understand. Some services are eligible only to those individuals who have specific disabilities, are of certain ages, or reside in particular localities. Services are offered at only designated times of the day or year, and have specific procedures as to eligibility, referral, registration, and payment. Problems thus arise in knowing about, understanding, becoming eligible for, paying for, and accessing such services. The web can help in accessing disability services—and parents and individuals with disabilities do use the web to access information and services (Zaidman-Zait & Jamieson, 2007)—but the effectiveness of web-only procedures remains unclear.

Partly to alleviate this problem, various human-service domains have developed information-and-referral (or I&R) services. Broadly stated, I&R services have the goal of helping people to find and use human services. I&R services also have a main professional organization, the Alliance of Information and Referral Systems (AIRS), that has 5000 members and is affiliated with over 1200 U.S. I&R agencies (described more below).

To quote the AIRS website, "Information and Referral (I&R) is the art, science and practice of bringing people and services together. When individuals and families don't know where to turn, I&R is there for them" (AIRS, 2018).

In considering disability services for individuals and their families, now may be an especially important time for the development of I&R services. As we document below, the past few decades have seen a proliferation of individual services; even faced with economic uncertainty and with state and federal governments that often de-value such services, the numbers and types of disability services are growing. At the same time, disability services are like sprouting weeds—multiplying and growing, but also uncoordinated, going off in multiple directions. It is therefore not enough for diverse services to exist, especially if potential recipients do not know about many services or cannot determine which services are most appropriate, whether a particular individual is eligible, or how to sign up for and receive the service. Individuals with IDD, their families, and providers may thus constitute the perfect targets of I&R, "the art, science and practice of bringing people and services together."

In the pages that follow, we discuss I&R services as they apply to individuals with intellectual and developmental disabilities. We begin by describing the many types of disability services, before discussing key components of information sciences more generally and of I&R services for individuals with disabilities and their families. Finally, after describing one such I&R service, Tennessee Disability Pathfinder, we discuss challenges in developing such services and ties of disability I&R services to ongoing service and policy initiatives.

1. DISABILITY SERVICES IN THE UNITED STATES: MANY WEEDS SPROUTING

Many families, individuals, and professionals hold the view that few services exist for individuals with disabilities. This perception likely arises from the scattered, uncoordinated nature of disability service systems and the way in which many disability services remain unknown to the general public. Also contributing to perceptions of scarcity are the ways in which services and access to services vary across and within states. Our discussion also focuses primarily on disability services in the United States; other industrialized countries have similar (albeit not identical) service systems (for examples, see Hatton, 2017; Roberts et al., 2018; Wark, Hussain, & Edwards, 2014).

In delving more deeply into American disability-related services, we discover a more complicated state of affairs. Across the United States, there exists a wide array of disability-related services and service systems. Included here are government-run and private services; services focused on infants, children, and young, middle-aged, and older adults; and service domains that range across early intervention and education, to health and mental health, to Supplemental Security Income (SSI) and Social Security Disability Insurance (SSDI), to post-secondary education and employment, to transportation and housing, to parent- and family support, to arts, leisure, sports, and other community-based activities. Some services are available to individuals with all disabilities, others to those with intellectual and developmental disabilities or with a specific type or cause of intellectual disability (e.g., Down syndrome, autism, cerebral palsy). Many professions also have sub-groups that specialize in the care of children or adults with disabilities (e.g., developmental pediatrics; psychiatric social work), and a few also have allied organizations or special interest groups (SIGs) within larger professional organizations (e.g., Division 33, on Intellectual and Developmental Disabilities and Autism Spectrum Disorders, within the larger American Psychological Association).

1.1 Description of Services

To document this array of services across the United States, Table 1 provides a quick overview. The table is divided into domains such as education, health, law, adult services, employment, early intervention, family support (siblings), recreation and leisure; disability organizations; assistive technology; and respite. For each entry, we provide the: (1) Name of organization; (2) Year founded; (3) How to access this organization; (4) Number of chapters/offices and membership size (if known); and (5) What the organization does.

In considering this table, a few points deserve mention. First, as extensive as Table 1 may seem, this listing is admittedly incomplete. We have not attempted in this paper to track down the many local services, or the current initiatives and projects of local chapters of these larger organizations. We have also not attempted to discover the many clinics, outreach efforts, camps, pilot or demonstration projects, or other initiatives that are currently occurring across the country. In addition to the organizations/departments listed in the table, such local initiatives also provide help and support to individuals with IDD and their families.

Second, this list does not highlight the ways in which disability services are linked within multiple networks. Among federally funded services, the

Table 1 Prominent Disability-Related Services Across the United States

Type	Organization	Start	How to Access	Chapters/Members	What They Do
Education	Early Intervention	1986	Contact Early Intervention District Office and ask for a developmental screening.	50+ state dept's, each w/lead agency	Provides family-centered interventions that focus on enhancing the development of children with disabilities from 0–3 years of age in hopes of minimizing their potential for developmental delays.
	Special Education	1975	All public schools are required by law to provide special education services to eligible students with a disability.	State dept's & Local Ed Agencies per district	Provides an individualized education to students 3–22 years old with a disability who qualify under one or more of the 13 eligibility categories.
	Special Education Advocacy Training (SEAT) www.copaa.org/?SEAT	2005	Individuals can register for courses via the Council of Parent Attorneys and Advocates website.	National training course	Year-long training course for participants to become special education advocates, offered as a combination of self-paced web learning, readings, group and individual assignments, and live virtual classrooms.

(Continued)

Table 1 Prominent Disability-Related Services Across the United States—cont'd

Type	Organization	Start	How to Access	Chapters/Members	What They Do
	Council for Exceptional Children (CEC) www.cec.sped.org	1922	Individuals can apply for membership on the CEC website.	48 state chapters	Professional association of educators dedicated to advancing the success of children with exceptionalities through advocacy, standards, and professional development.
Health	Leadership Education in Neurodevelopmental and related Disabilities (LEND) www.aucd.org/template/page.cfm?id=473	1950s	Contact local LEND program to determine how to become involved.	52 programs across 44 states	Provides interdisciplinary training, have faculty and trainees in a wide range of disciplines, and include parents or family members as paid program participants.
	American Academy of Developmental Medicine and Dentistry www.aadmd.org	2002	Individuals can apply for membership on their website.	National organization	Provides a forum for healthcare professionals who provide clinical care to people with neurodevelopmental disorders and intellectual disabilities in order to improve the quality of healthcare for these populations.

Society for Developmental and Behavioral Pediatrics www.sdbp.org	1982	Individuals can apply for membership on their website.	National organization	Improves the health care of infants, children, and adolescents by promoting research and teaching in developmental and behavioral pediatrics.
Healthy Athletes Program of Special Olympics International	1997	Participants contact local-state-national branch of Special Olympics International	National (& international) organization	Provides health exams & education (often at local-state-national Special Olympics events) in 7 areas: general fitness, podiatry, hearing, vision, dental hygiene, healthy lifestyle choices, & sports physicals.
American Academy for Cerebral Palsy and Developmental Medicine www.aacpdm.org	1947	Participants from all disciplines that work with children with cerebral palsy and other developmental disabilities can apply on the website.	National organization	Provides multidisciplinary scientific education for health professionals and promotes excellence in research and services for people with cerebral palsy and other childhood-onset disabilities.

(Continued)

Table 1 Prominent Disability-Related Services Across the United States—cont'd

Type	Organization	Start	How to Access	Chapters/Members	What They Do
	Developmental Disabilities Nurses Association www.ddna.org	1992	Nurses who work with children and adults with developmental disabilities can apply on the organization's website.	31 chapters	Nursing organization committed to advocacy, education, and support for nurses who provide services to persons with intellectual and developmental disabilities.
	Down Syndrome Clinics www.globaldownsyndrome.org/research-medical-care/medical-care-providers/	Varies	Individuals can find local clinic on website.	Clinics in 33 states ($\approx$60 total)	Medical clinics that specialize in treating patients with Down syndrome.
Law	Fragile X Clinics www.fragilex.org/research/#1498268491073-e38da661-8aca	Varies	Individuals can find a local clinic on their website.	31 clinics across 22 states	Medical clinics that specialize in treating patients with Fragile X syndrome.
	Protection and Advocacy for Individuals with Developmental Disabilities www.ndrn.org/about/paacap-network.html	1975	Individuals with a disability or their family members can contact their local state P&A agency to request legal or advocacy services.	57 chapters	Pursues legal, administrative and other appropriate remedies to protect and advocate for the rights of individuals with developmental disabilities.

Council of Parent Attorneys and Advocates (COPAA) http://copaa.site-ym.com/	1998	Families can find local advocates using the online directory on their website.	National organization	Protects and enforces the legal and civil rights of students with disabilities and their families, primarily through securing high quality educational services and promoting excellence in advocacy.
National Center on Criminal Justice and Disability (NCCJD) www.thearc.org/NCCJD	2013	A form is available on their website to request legal assistance.	National organization	Works to build the capacity of the criminal justice system to respond to gaps in existing services for people with disabilities, specifically focusing on people with intellectual and developmental disabilities.
Parent Training and Information Centers (PTIs) www.parentcenterhub.org/find-your-center	1983	Contact local chapter. Information can be found on the Center for Parent Information and Resources website.	64 (at least one per state)	Provides no-cost assistance to families on how to navigate special education services.

(*Continued*)

Table 1 Prominent Disability-Related Services Across the United States—cont'd

Type	Organization	Start	How to Access	Chapters/Members	What They Do
Adult Services	Volunteer Advocacy Project www.vkc.mc.vanderbilt.edu/vkc/services/project/volunteer-advocacy	2008	Applications to participate can be found on website. Advocates who graduated from the program can also be requested.	Primary training center with satellite locations (TN, IL, KY)	Trains interested individuals to become special education advocates so they can provide instrumental and affective support to families of children with disabilities.
	Councils on Developmental Disabilities www.nacdd.org	2000	Locate local state chapter on website.	50+ state chapters (& PR and territories)	Independent state agencies that work to ensure that people with developmental disabilities receive the services and supports they need that promote self-determination, integration, and inclusion.
	Department of Developmental Disability www.nasddds.org/state-agencies/	Early 1960s	Locate state agencies on website.	50 state chapters (& PR and territories)	Independent state agencies that work to develop effective, efficient service delivery to children and adults with intellectual and developmental disabilities and their families.

Employment	Aging and Disability Resource Centers (ADRC's) www.acl.gov/programs/aging-and-disability-networks/aging-and-disability-resource-centers	2003	Find local chapter to determine what services are available.	50 state chapters (& PR and territories)	Provides objective information, advice, counseling and assistance; empowers people to make informed decisions about their long-term services and supports; and helps people access public and private programs.
	Employer Assistance and Resource Network on Disability Inclusion (EARN) www.askearn.org	2015	All resources are available for free online.	National organization	Provides free resources that help employers recruit, hire, and retain employees with disabilities
Family Support-Parents/Siblings	Vocational Rehabilitation	1973	Contact local VR office to determine eligibility.	50 state chapters (& PR and territories)	Federal-state program that works with individuals with disabilities to develop an Individualized Plan for Employment (IPE) which outlines a program of services that leads to successful employment.

(Continued)

Table 1 Prominent Disability-Related Services Across the United States—cont'd

Type	Organization	Start	How to Access	Chapters/Members	What They Do
	Sibling Leadership Network www.siblingleadership.org	2007	Individuals can apply for membership on their website.	25 chapters	Provides siblings of individuals with disabilities the information, support, and tools to advocate with their brothers and sisters and to promote the issues important to them and their entire families.
	Sibling Support Project www. siblingsupport.org	1990	Individuals can use the online directory on their website to find a sibshop near them.	475 sibshops across 8 countries	Provides opportunities for siblings of individuals with disabilities to connect with other siblings and access peer support in a variety of settings.
	National Down Syndrome Congress (NDSC) https://www.ndsccenter.org/	1973	View information on website, Can join by becoming a member or an affiliate program subscriber, Can support through donations.	National organization	Leading national resource of support and information about Down Syndrome. Promotes interests of people with Down Syndrome and their families through advocacy, public awareness, and information.

Recreation and Leisure	Autism Society of America (ASA) http://www.autism-society.org/	1965	Information found on website, National Contact Center phone line, hosts annual national conference	National organization	Provide advocacy, education, information and referral, support, and community at national, state, and local levels through their strong nationwide network of Affiliates.
	The International Organization on Arts and Disability (VSA) www.education.kennedy-center.org/education/vsa	1974	Contact local affiliate chapter to find opportunities to get involved.	52 int. affiliates & network of nationwide affiliates	Provides individuals with disabilities access to high quality arts learning experiences.
	Special Olympics www.specialolympics.org	1968	Individuals with intellectual disabilities over 2 years old can register to participate by contacting their local chapter.	54 state chapters (& PR and territories)	Provides year-round sports training and athletic competition in a variety of Olympic-type sports for children and adults with intellectual disabilities.
Disability Organizations	National Arts and Disability Center (NADC) www.semel.ucla.edu/nadc	1984	Individuals with disabilities can apply for the Arts and Accessibility Technical Assistance Program on website.	National center	Promotes the full inclusion of audiences and artists with disabilities into all facets of the arts community.

(Continued)

Table 1 Prominent Disability-Related Services Across the United States—cont'd

Type	Organization	Start	How to Access	Chapters/Members	What They Do
	University Centers of Excellence in Developmental Disabilities (UCEDD) www.aucd.org/template/page.cfm?id=24	1963	Contact local UCEDD to determine opportunities to get involved.	50+ state chapters (& PR and territories)	Supports interdisciplinary training, services, research, and dissemination of information in the field of developmental disabilities.
	The Arc www.thearc.org	1950s	Interested individuals, including self-advocates, family members, professionals in the field, and others, can become a member on the Arc's website.	730 local chapters across 39 states	Promotes and protects the human rights of people with intellectual and developmental disabilities through the use of various programs, training opportunities, and additional resources.
	National Down Syndrome Society (NDSS) www.ndss.org	1980s	Access website to find local Buddy Walk and determine ways to get involved in state- or national-level advocacy.	National organization	Advocates for the human rights of individuals with Down syndrome.
	Autism Speaks www.autismspeaks.org	2005	Families can find autism-related resources on the website or get involved by participating in a local event or fundraiser.	National organization	Promotes solutions, across the spectrum and throughout the lifespan, for the needs of individuals with autism and their families.

Assistive Technology	United Cerebral Palsy www.ucp.org	1949	Families can contact their local UCP affiliate to determine available services.	National organization, 65 UCP Affiliates	Advocates for and provides services to adults and children with disabilities through the use of their affiliate network.
Respite	State Assistive Technology Programs www.ataporg.org	1998	Individuals with disabilities can access assistive technology by contacting their local state chapter.	50 state chapters (& PR and territories)	Teaches individuals with disabilities, service providers and others about assistive technology (AT) needed for education, employment, and community living.
	ARCH National Respite Network www.archrespite.org	1990	Families can use the website to search for Respite programs and resources in their state.	22 chapters across 22 states	Promotes the development of quality respite and crisis care programs in the United States and helps families locate respite and crisis care services in their communities.

67 University Centers of Excellence in Developmental Disabilities, or UCEDD's, provide disability-related service and outreach, training, research, and dissemination in each of the 50 states and most US territories (AUCD, 2012a). Beyond the work of each UCEDD itself, these UCEDD's are organized into a larger national network. This larger network holds an annual national conference, disseminates frequent e-mails and newsletters, and directs a national reporting system of all projects and activities occurring in each UCEDD (NIRS, the National Information Reporting System). The UCEDD network also features sub-groups and coalitions on specific topics (e.g., employment, post-secondary education, religion, research, families).

Within the AUCD network, there are also sub-networks that are more specifically focused on pre-professional training and on research support. Thus, a national network occurs with the country's 52 Leadership Education in Neurodevelopmental and Related Disabilities, or LEND, programs (AUCD, 2012b). This one-year long program, housed in multiple universities and medical centers across the country, introduces students in 12 (mostly medically-oriented) fields about disabilities, the US disability-service system, and using multi-disciplinary teams to treat individuals with disabilities. The AUCD network also includes the 14 Eunice Kennedy Shriver-Intellectual and Developmental Disability Research Centers (EKS-IDDRCs). These EKS-IDDRCs provide administrative, statistical, recruitment, biophysical (e.g., MRI's, EEGs) and other support for human and non-human (e.g. mouse model) disability-related research. The UCEDDs, LENDs, and IDDRCs all come under the umbrella of the Association of University Centers on Disabilities (or AUCD; www.aucd.org). But other national networks are also active, including approximately 64 Parent Training and Information Centers, which train parents on their special education rights (PTIs; www.parentcenterhub.org), the 57 (legal) Protection and Advocacy organizations (P&As; organized under the National Disability Rights Network) in each state (www.ndrn.org), and the National Association of Councils on Developmental Disabilities, with its "DD Councils" which coordinate disability initiatives in each state (56 overall; https://nacdd.org).

Beyond these federally-funded initiatives, many large-scale private organizations also exist. The two most prominent are The Arc and organizations of the Joseph P. Kennedy, Jr. Foundation. The (national) Arc has 730 individual chapters, with statewide chapters and (in some states) multiple county or city-town chapters. Funded by member dues, private philanthropy and grants, The Arc describes itself as the "leading advocate for all people with intellectual and developmental disabilities and their families and the premier provider of the supports and services that people need." In addition to The Arc, several organizations of the Joseph P. Kennedy, Jr. Foundation—most notably Special Olympics, Best Buddies, and VSA (formerly, Very Special Arts)—also have state and local chapters, thousands of volunteers, and programs in sports, companionship-friendship, and arts (respectively) that serve large numbers of individuals with disabilities.

1.2 History

Table 1 also only hints at the rich history of the services themselves, as both the advocates for and recipients of societal change. Consider one major organization, The Arc. Founded in 1950, The Arc boasts the leading role that it played in the deinstitutionalization movement and in advocating for PL 94−142, the 1975 federal law ensuring a free, appropriate public education for all US schoolchildren (http://www.thearc.org/who-we-are/history/advocacy). Indeed, the main "right to education" court case leading to PL 94−142, PARC v. Commonwealth of Pennsylvania, featured as the named litigant the Pennsylvania chapter of the ARC (see https://www.youtube.com/watch?v=QtFmp3XduaQ for the chapter's role in the PARC lawsuit).

Moving in the opposite direction, many federal initiatives have led to (and continue to foster) services for individuals with disabilities and their families. Most prominent here are the actions and outgrowths of the John F. Kennedy administration. Spurred on by the tireless efforts of his sister, Eunice Kennedy Shriver, President Kennedy in 1961 called for the establishment of the first President's Committee on Mental Retardation, or PCMR. In surveying the country's efforts, that blue-ribbon committee discovered a primitive, inadequate state of affairs in outreach and services, training, and research in intellectual disabilities (Shorter, 2000). The PCMR report, in turn, led to the establishment of the 67 UCEDDs providing disability-related outreach and services, the 52 LENDs providing inter-disciplinary disability training to pre-professional students in 12 mostly medically oriented disciplines; and the 14 EKS-IDDRCs supporting inter-disciplinary IDD research—together, the UCEDDs, LENDs, and EKS-IDDRCs now constitute the infrastructure of modern-day service, training, and research in intellectual disabilities (Hodapp, Fidler, & Depta, 2016). Summarizing such advances, the historian Edward Berkowitz (1980) concluded that, in contrast to many initiatives started but left unfinished during the Kennedy administration, in the area of intellectual disabilities, "the Kennedy Administration could claim that this triumph was theirs, all theirs" (p. 142).

1.3 Disorganized and Uncoordinated Services

Table 1's listing of disability services is impressive, especially in its numbers and types of different services. At the same time, however, this array of organizations/departments remains scattered and uncoordinated. Granted, some degree of organization does exist, mostly within state or local centers or chapters of a single organization. The 67 UCEDDs are grouped together, as are the 64 PTIs and 56 DD Councils. Within private disability organizations, the many local or state chapters of organizations such as Special Olympics, The Arc, or United Cerebral Palsy are linked with their respective larger, national organizations. Many such networks exist within disability services.

Overall, though, the general pattern is one of scattered, uncoordinated services. Especially when crossing categories—when simultaneously considering (for instance) disability-related clinics (e.g., medical clinics in Down syndrome) and arts or recreation programs (e.g., state or local VSA or Best Buddies chapters)—one sees few connections. In addition, locations differ for particular services. Services are also unequally spread out within a state by type of profession; for example, even compared to the home-office locations of Speech Language Pathologists (SLP's) throughout one state (Tennessee), that state's Board Certified Behavior Analysts (BCBA's) were disproportionally located in or near cities, much less often in the state's rural areas (Mello, Goldman, Urbano, & Hodapp, 2016). Further complications arise given inconsistency of names: in Tennessee, the Parent Training and Intervention Centers—or PTIs—are known as STEP (Support and Training for Exceptional Parents), with the main statewide office in Greeneville (in East Tennessee), and satellite offices in the state's Middle (Nashville) and West (Memphis) regions. Although the issue of differing names has begun to be addressed—note the recent movement of the (legal-oriented) Protection and Advocacy (P&A) to all adopt the name "Disability Rights [STATE NAME]"—the problem remains for certain groups and in certain states.

A final complication concerns the degree to which services wax and wane over time. Here we focus not on the larger organizations, but on their new initiatives. Especially for the many organizations listed in Table 1, new initiatives are common at the national, state, or local level, with such initiatives often supported by governmental or private foundation grant funding.

In most cases, such funding lasts for only three or five years. After that time, funding ends, paid staff look elsewhere for employment, and services, clinical trials, or interventions end. As a result, a continuous coming-and-going ensues, with many helpful, effective disability services existing for several years, after which time the service disappears.

There are, then, many disability-related services, but such services are difficult to understand and put together. Prospective users of such services require help in identifying which services currently exist, where a particular service is located, whether one is eligible for the service, and (if so) how one registers for, pays for, and receives the service. As a result, individuals with disabilities, their parents, their families, and professionals all become perfect recipients of Information and Referral services.

2. INFORMATION MOVEMENT IN LIBRARY SCIENCE AND I&R SERVICES

When we contemplate the information revolution, we often think of computers and computer science. As a society, we revel in the stories of Steve Jobs and Steve Wozniak creating the Apple I computer in Jobs' garage, and of Bill Gates dropping out of Harvard to sell his operating system for IBM's new personal computer, thus ensuring that Microsoft would thrive over the next 50 years.

2.1 The Information Revolution and Library Sciences

But on a practical level, the information revolution encompasses three different areas: computer science, telecommunications, and library science (Yan, 2011). Of these, the most important for the current discussion is library science, especially library science's increasing focus on information as opposed to books and libraries. As computer science developed over the mid- and late-20th century, the field of library sciences followed suit: Yan (2011) notes that, after about the year 2000, most Library Science departments renamed themselves departments or schools of Information Sciences or Library and Information Sciences; from the 1970s through 1990s, over 10 introductory texts were published on this now-revised discipline.

Beyond these changes in name, four content changes were also occurring (Rubin, 2004). First, the field explicitly focused on information, regardless of package (book, database) or context (government, business, personal). Library sciences thus moved "away from the book to information itself" (p. 33).

Second, librarians—now better considered as information science professionals—focused on the entire information cycle, from creation to use, and involving acquiring, organizing, maintaining, and disseminating such information. Third, the field became increasingly inter-disciplinary, relying heavily on computer science for advances in computer-user interfaces and on cognitive psychology for understandings of how users search for, gather, evaluate, and use information.

Fourth, the library and information science field focused on the accessibility and usability of information. This movement emphasized both the contexts underlying the need for information and the individual's potential uses of that information. As Durrance (1989) noted, the issue became not only "What do you want to know?" but also "How and why is the information needed? How is it likely to help? What does the user know already? What is expected? What are the parameters of the problem?" (p. 163).

2.2 Information and Referral (I&R) Services

Given the changing nature of library and information sciences—as well as the changing roles of librarians themselves—the development of I&R services seems almost predetermined. One could argue that I&R services merely expanded the traditional role of the reference librarian. In prior years, that librarian sat at a desk and fielded queries from library patrons. With I&R services, that core mission has expanded to providing information that helps the user access needed social services.

Though earlier initiatives occurred in both the US and Great Britain, the first modern attempts to develop I&R services began in the 1960s and 1970s. During that time, three agencies—the United Way of America (UWA), the Administration on Aging (AoA), and the Alliance of Information and Referral Systems (AIRS)—worked together to foster the growth of American I&R services. Levinson (2002) refers to these three national organizations as the National I&R Triad (p. 8).

Although a more extensive history is beyond the scope of this chapter, the National I&R Triad figures prominently in many of the field's key events:

- 1973—Older Americans Act (OAA)–states should develop and maintain I&R services (the original Older Americans Act of 1965 stipulated that information, referral, and assistance are required to help older adults remain in their own homes and communities; Levinson, 2002);
- 1973—founding of Alliance of Information and Referral Systems (AIRS). AIRS continues to be the main professional organization of

information-and-referral services, promulgating I&R standards; overseeing training, accreditation, and professional certifications for I&R providers; overseeing terminology and taxonomy of terms; organizing professional conferences, workshops, and newsletters; promulgating ethical standards for I&R providers; and acting "as a seal of approval for organizations providing community I&R services, so funders can confidently identify and support providers that create the community impact they seek" (www.airs.org).

- 1983—AIRS and United Way update original (1973) standards and publish study indicating that approximately 80% of all I&R services in the US were designed specifically for older persons;
- 1988—National Association of States United for Aging and Disabilities (NASUAD)—performs feasibility study recommending establishing a national toll-free access system;
- 1990—U.S. Administration on Aging—begins two-pronged I&R initiative involving Eldercare Locator and National Aging I&R/A (i.e. Information and Referral/Assistance) Support Centers.
- 2000—Federal Communications Commission (FCC) reserves 2-1-1-dialing code for community I&R services. First begun in Connecticut in 1998–99, as of February 2015 these 2-1-1 lines served over 291 million Americans, covering all or parts of 50 states, as well as Washington, DC and Puerto Rico (helplinecenter.org, 2017).
- 2003—start of Aging and Disability Resource Centers (ADRCs), which now include 56 state agencies (including DC and territories), 622 area agencies on aging, and 260 Title VI Native American aging programs. Although concerns remain about whether ADRCs adequately meet the needs of aging adults with disabilities (Coyle, Putman, Kramer, & Mutchler, 2016), this network attempts to provide "one-stop shopping" for services for aging adults and aging adults with disabilities;
- Past decade—Network-wide movement toward integrating aging and disability service-delivery systems.

Given these brief histories of library-information science and of I&R services, we now describe the components of I&R services. Although differing in content and scope, I&R services—especially those that are "more client-centered" (Levinson, 2002)—generally show the following six characteristics (Community Ambassadors Providing for Services, CAPS, 2017):

(1) *Understanding people's situations.* Whether in disabilities, aging, or other content area, I&R services begin by understanding the person's individual situation. Especially given the complexity of disability-related services, staff members of disability-related I&R services need to understand the age, home location, disability type and severity, family situation, services currently received, and recent service history of the person with disabilities. The original reason for the query is important, but serves only as the initial starting point. As conversations continue, seasoned I&R workers discover other (sometimes less obvious) issues, identify other unmet service needs, and consider additional programs or initiatives for which the person and his/her family may be eligible.

(2) *Providing clients with resources.* Client-centered I&R services are not hypothetical or theoretical; they are practical. Clients receive information that is individualized, current, and helpful. In response to a call from a mother seeking services for her 2-year old child with autism, the disability I&R worker tells the mother about that particular state's early intervention system, the way in which services are provided until 3 years of age (after which school-based services commence), how testing and assessments will proceed and how eligibility will be determined, and how (if eligible) the child, mother, and family will receive in-home or center-based services.

In addition to such background information, however, the mother will be provided practical facts. She will be told where the EI system's nearest office is located, what the phone number and the web address are, and sometimes even who to speak with and what to request. For callers needing more assistance, the information provider might talk through with the mother how to describe her child and the child's condition, what kinds of documentation might be necessary, and how specific problems or functioning levels might be described. The caller is provided with practical resources and strategies that can be used in subsequent attempts to access services.

(3) *Prioritizing and planning.* As service systems are bureaucratic, the information providers of an I&R service also need to prioritize activities in asking for services. For the mother of the 2-year old with autism, it would be inefficient to begin by calling a local service provider of, say, speech-language services. Unless the mother was insistent on going to the local speech-language therapist for private therapy (paid for by the family), that mother may first need to contact the people who oversee the child's entry into the early intervention system, the state's "lead agency" devoted to early intervention, which differs by state. In speaking with these people, the mother can then provide information on the child and family and the child can be scheduled for testing and diagnosis. Only later, after such testing has been completed, would the state's early intervention system approve that child's speech-language and other services. In addition to the ordering and timing of events, seasoned I&R professionals will also alert the mother to any necessary documents or forms to begin the process.

(4) *Identifying and understanding community resources.* To serve clients in the best way possible, disability I&R information-providers must be knowledgeable. To access services for an individual with Down syndrome, for example, the information provider must be aware of health conditions that often co-occur during childhood, such things as heart defects, respiratory problems, celiac disease, and leukemia (Roizen, 2010). Middle-aged adults with Down syndrome often also face issues with Alzheimer's dementia (Zigman, 2013) and may, due to more often having older parents and more often living in the family home, require that the family receive extra assistance in caregiving (Hodapp, Burke, Finley, & Hodapp, 2016).

Information providers must also have good understandings of current disability services. Some of this knowledge relates to a specific condition—for example, approximately 60 Down syndrome clinics are located across the United States (see Table 1; see also the website of the National Organization of Rare Disorders; NORD, 2018). Other critical knowledge concerns how disability services work, with most services differing from the 0–3 year period (the time of state-run early intervention services), to the 3–22 year period, when most education-related services are under the aegis of local school districts, to the adult years, when residential, work, waiver, and other services exist, but often with different eligibility criteria (and, in many states, long waiting lists). These different ages of service also feature policies, regulations, and laws that change over time. Recently, for example, Tennessee passed a law mandating that adults with disabilities would hereafter be removed from waiting lists and qualified to receive state disability services when they lived at home and were cared for by parents and caregivers who were older than 80 years of age. This new state policy would naturally become part of any service conversation for elderly parents calling about services for their adult offspring.

(5) *When necessary, advocating.* As members of their local disability communities, disability I&R information providers have long histories of dealing with service providers. In addition to providing information and, at times, offering strategies for whom and how to approach other agencies, these staff members will sometimes directly advocate for individuals or families who they serve. Granted, such direct advocacy may best be conceptualized as a last resort. Still, if they are to reach their goal of linking individuals and families with appropriate services, direct advocacy may sometimes be necessary.

(6) *Following-up*. To link people with services, it is not enough to meet or speak with someone, provide information and strategies, and say goodbye. Seasoned I&R professionals appreciate that individuals with disabilities and their family members are entering a different world, a world with which the caller may be totally or partially unfamiliar. Follow-up contacts are therefore critical to determine whether the client persevered until making contact with the relevant disability-service agency. If not, the I&R staff member needs to find out what happened, talk through additional steps, and negotiate a revised plan of action.

2.3 Issues Pertaining to Disability I&R Information Providers

In considering the many characteristics of I&R services, one can sense just how difficult it is to provide good disability I&R services. Many of these difficulties relate to the personal and professional qualities needed by I&R service providers, a subject to which we now turn.

The clinically-sensitive role of the disability I&R information-provider. More than simply providing information, effective disability I&R staff members find out more about the needs, issues, and perspectives of the clients with whom they are dealing. In the case of disability I&R services, such issues often relate to two parties: parents or other family members and the person with disabilities (although adults with disabilities often directly use disability I&R services). The topics of discussion are sensitive in that they relate to the need for help—itself a sensitive issue—and to health, mental health, need for financial assistance, living or work situation, or other personal matters of the individual with a disability and parents.

In dealing with these issues, the disability I&R information provider must have good clinical skills. Although variously defined, clinical skills include the ability to listen carefully, to clarify what the client is saying, to communicate clearly, to be empathetic and non-judgmental, and to engage jointly with the client in some type of problem-solving. In this context, the information provider must also be able to listen closely to the client, clarify which services are needed, and probe to find out at which point the client is in the process of knowing about, requesting, and accessing needed services.

Each activity must be done in as non-judgmental a fashion as possible, with careful attention to the age, gender, cultural and linguistic background, and understandings of the person requesting help.

Although information-providers use many clinical skills when providing I&R services, the most prominent may involve "active" or "therapeutic" listening. Long considered a hallmark of effective mental health services (Rogers, 1957; Watanuki, Tracy, & Lindquist, 2014), active listening includes both non-verbal and verbal behaviors. Non-verbal behaviors, which are needed during face-to-face meetings, include high levels of eye contact, appropriate head nods, facial pleasantness, forward leans, body orientation toward the client, open body orientation, appropriate smiling, animation, and vocal pleasantness. Verbal behaviors are needed for any type of conversation; examples are asking open-ended questions, paraphrasing the client's statements, reflecting feelings, and explicitly checking out assumptions (Bodie, Vickery, Cannava, & Jones, 2015). Such non-verbal and verbal techniques can be taught to untrained individuals; when used, these techniques seem effective in fostering the client's feelings that the provider has been helpful, sensitive, and supportive (Bodie, et al., 2015).

But the I&R professional is also not a trained or certified mental health, health, or allied health provider. They should not provide diagnoses of any type, including speculations as to a client's health condition, psychiatric diagnosis, or genetic syndrome. Nor should the information-provider make therapeutic recommendations (including the use of herbal remedies) or give psychological counseling. Such warnings are explicitly noted in guidelines concerning the appropriate roles of I&R providers (CAPS, 2017). Suspecting that a problem may exist, I&R professionals may refer the client to a mental health professional, physician, or clinical geneticist, but they should keep their more specific suspicions to themselves.

Another sensitive issue concerns the balance between empowering individuals to gain services versus directly providing individuals with a service. Here we invoke the old Chinese adage: "Give someone a fish and you feed them for a day. Teach them how to fish and you feed them for a lifetime." Although the stated goal of all I&R services is to bring "people and services together" (AIRS, 2018), receiving services sometimes conflicts with empowering the client. To the extent possible, disability-related I&R services should encourage clients to themselves request services. The implicit goal is to empower the client to access services, both by becoming more comfortable psychologically and by gaining practical knowledge and experience. Such gains in comfort and in knowledge have long been considered important when working with parents of offspring with disabilities, and can also be positively affected by specific interventions (Burke, Goldman, Hart, & Hodapp, 2016; Taylor, Hodapp, Burke, Waitz-Kudla, & Rabideau, 2017). Such goals are contrasted by the fact that disability services are indeed difficult to negotiate and, in many cases, the I&R professionals have good relationships with the relevant service agency or provider. Why not just make the calls themselves?

In most instances, such a decision would be unwise. It is generally not good practice for disability I&R professionals to do too much for the client asking for information. Keeping in mind the dual goal of attaining services and empowering the client, the information provider might instead teach or model how to access services. Teaching might involve providing the client more information about the principles of the disability-service system, for instance that services are directed by state agencies during early childhood (0–3 EI services) and adulthood (age 21+), whereas 3–21 year old services are directed by local school districts. Modeling or role-playing may also come into play when the information provider demonstrates what to say when making a call to a state agency or school district. Although teaching or modeling somewhat extends beyond providing information, in most cases such practices should suffice for parents and individuals with disabilities to navigate their local disability service system.

Ultimately, as disability-related I&R services are finite, parents and individuals must advocate for themselves. Granted, such advocacy efforts may be difficult; require the combined efforts of parents, siblings, and individuals with disabilities; and change over the lifespan (Burke et al., 2016). Disability I&R specialists will sometimes be tempted to do the work themselves, to phone or email other disability professionals. That tendency, however, needs to be balanced by the knowledge that I&R resources are limited, that extraordinary efforts may not prove cost-effective, and that a secondary goal of I&R services concerns developing the client's own skills. One wants the client to receive the fish—the appropriate services—but one also wants the client to learn how to fish (and to become comfortable fishing), how to navigate disability service systems on their own.

The importance of being a disability insider. In recent years, various researchers have expressed concern as to the extent to which samples in disability-family research reflect the larger population of families of individuals with disabilities. Whereas studies using population-based records find that families of individuals with disabilities are disproportionately of low socioeconomic status and from minority groups (Fujiura, 2014), many studies using so-called samples of convenience discover that their family samples are disproportionately White, middle-class, and well-educated. It remains unclear the degree to which the issues and concerns of such groups reflect the larger population of families of offspring with disabilities (Magaña, Seltzer, & Krauss, 2004; Parish, Rose, & Swaine, 2010).

Another concern relates to the degree to which any research participant is a part of the local disability community. Oftentimes, families hear about a study by belonging to a disability organization. Many of these individuals receive disability-organization newsletters or email alerts; belong to listservs, chat rooms, or other social media related to disabilities; count among their personal friends other parents or siblings of persons with disabilities; and/ or spend their time working for disability-related organizations, events, or initiatives. They are disability insiders. This degree to which research participants are connected to the world of disability might be another, mostly unexamined, way in which the samples of many studies may not represent the wider population of families of persons with disabilities (Sanderson, Burke, Urbano, Arnold, & Hodapp, 2017).

Though a challenge from a research perspective, being a disability insider may constitute a necessary prerequisite for a disability I&R information provider. To know, for example, which grant-supported disability services are currently active, one needs to know the local disability field, its people, and its organizations. For this reason, the Tennessee Disability Pathfinder service (discussed below) frequently updates its listing of services and organizations. Pathfinder staff appreciate the importance of staying current, that a service or local affiliate that existed even 6 months ago may now be inactive or defunct. In the same way, the information provider must be aware of new state initiatives, for example, the change in Tennessee law to place offspring of elderly caregiving parents onto the waiver. Only an information provider who is "in the know" would appreciate the implications of this change in state law.

3. EXAMPLE OF A DISABILITY I&R SERVICE: TENNESSEE DISABILITY PATHFINDER

To make more concrete many of the issues discussed above, we describe one disability-related I&R service, Tennessee Disability Pathfinder. Run as a long-term partnership between the Tennessee Council on Developmental Disabilities (TN DD Council) and the Vanderbilt Kennedy

Center, we begin by presenting Pathfinder's history, then highlight some of the service's main characteristics and changes.

3.1 The History of Tennessee Disability Pathfinder

In 1996, the Tennessee Council on Developmental Disabilities identified the need for a statewide disability I&R service. In 1997, at the Council's annual strategic planning meeting, Council members agreed to create an I&R service that would serve all communities across Tennessee. Shortly thereafter, the Council Executive Director, Wanda Willis, met with then Kennedy Center Director Travis Thompson to invite the Kennedy Center to join as a partner with the Council in the endeavor. After discussions among key Center staff, the Kennedy Center enthusiastically accepted the Council's proposal to establish the Tennessee Disability Information and Referral Office (TDIR). The Council provided operational funds for the project and the Kennedy Center contributed matching costs and housed the project.

Initially staffed by a Project Coordinator (35 h/wk) and Assistant (20 h/wk), TDIR began on July 1, 1997. At that time, services included a local and toll-free helpline; a statewide community calendar of disability-related events created and maintained in collaboration with other Tennessee disability organizations; the creation of a database of disability-related services and social services from which directories would be published; community outreach; and quarterly evaluation of consumer and agency satisfaction. An Advisory Council was also established, with representation from Tennessee's three Grand Regions (West, Middle, East). The initial meeting of the Advisory Council took place in October 1997, with quarterly meetings thereafter. In 1998, TDIR first published three separate regional disability service directories for East, Middle, and West Tennessee, respectively.

Even within a short period of time, the newly-operational TDIR program was expanding and taking on new functions. In 2000, the Council received funding for a 2-year state Family Support project from the federal Administration on Developmental Disabilities [now Administration on Intellectual and Developmental Disabilities]. The Council contracted with the Kennedy Center to design and program the Tennessee Family Pathfinder as a gateway disability information website. The Council staff and members participated in each step of developing the website. With funds from the grant, the Kennedy Center and Council worked with a Nashville public relations firm [Dye, van Mol, and Lawrence] to conduct a statewide public awareness campaign. Quickly, Pathfinder became broadly known and well-used by families and agencies. Since Pathfinder and TDIR were interrelated, and since the Pathfinder website made the TDIR database searchable by the public, the two projects were unified in 2003–04. From that time forward, the service was named "Pathfinder," a continuing partnership of the Tennessee Council on Developmental Disabilities and the Vanderbilt Kennedy Center.

The federal Family Support grant also fostered an increased emphasis on reaching traditionally underserved populations. Specifically, the Council contracted with IAM CARES to create Leadership Institutes in the Nashville and Memphis Enterprise Communities for individuals with disabilities and family members who were African-American or Hispanic. At the same time, Pathfinder added a social worker who was bilingual in Spanish and English, whose role was outreach to Spanish-speaking communities across Tennessee. Pathfinder's commitment to connect Spanish-speaking families with disability services eventually led to the development of the Camino Seguro database and website, which included disability and social services provided by agencies that had bilingual staff. Camino Seguro began in Middle Tennessee through Pathfinder's collaboration with Nashville Metropolitan Social Services and the Mental Health Association of Middle Tennessee. In 2009, through a partnership with the University of Tennessee Boling Center for Developmental Disabilities and community partners, Camino Seguro expanded to West Tennessee. In 2010, it expanded as well to East Tennessee, again in partnership with community organizations. Today Camino Seguro is a single database maintained by Tennessee Disability Pathfinder.

In more recent years, Pathfinder's organization and services have expanded even further. In 2011, Pathfinder's Hispanic Outreach Program evolved to a Multicultural Outreach Program, inclusive of all cultures and languages. Over the years, Pathfinder has also hired staff members who have disabilities or have family members with disabilities, and staff from diverse cultures who are bilingual, e.g., Kurdish, Arabic. Today, Pathfinder's Multicultural Outreach Program includes a multilingual helpline, Camino Seguro, to link individuals with Spanish-speaking service providers, parent support groups, and disability and cultural awareness training and leadership of the Tennessee Multicultural Alliance on Disability.

3.2 Larger, Disability-Related I&R Themes

The history of Tennessee Disability Pathfinder highlights several important themes.

1) *Support of and collaboration with community partners.* Tennessee Disability Pathfinder involves a history of collaboration. From its initial days, when Tennessee's DD Council decided that it wanted to inaugurate this type of service, many organizations and agencies have been supportive. Members of the Advisory Council have devoted their time to ensuring that Pathfinder is working well and the state's other University Center for Excellence in Developmental Disabilities (UCEDD), the Boling Center for Developmental Disabilities at the University of Tennessee Health Sciences Center in Memphis, has been intimately involved in many of Pathfinder's expansions (especially its Camino Seguro project). Such organizational help has persisted over time and across the three grand regions of the state. Across its over two decades of operation, the Council has funded the majority of the initiative, at times along with other state of Tennessee or federal sources.

Such support—in terms of money, work, and interest—has helped bring together Tennessee's disability community. Anecdotally (and in contrast to some other states), Tennessee's many disability organizations work well together. Staff and members from different organizations often collaborate on joint projects; serve on disability-related advisory committees, blue-ribbon commissions, and organizational boards; know about, recruit for, and disseminate information about one another's events, initiatives, services, and social media campaigns; and help out in other ways. Disability-related events from Tennessee organizations appear on Pathfinder's web-calendar, as well as the Vanderbilt Kennedy Center's *Monday Morning Message*, a web-based newsletter e-mailed to 1700 individuals and organizations across the state. Obviously, this high level of cooperation is not solely due to Pathfinder's activities or efforts. But as a major part of the state's disability community, Pathfinder and its staff's efforts and activities deserve credit for helping to make the state's disability community more cohesive.

2) *Expansion over time.* Over its past 20 years, Tennessee Disability Pathfinder has expanded in numerous ways. First, Pathfinder has expanded in size. Originally managed by 1.5 staff members (i.e., one full-time & one half-time), Pathfinder has grown to six full-time and one part-time staff. Such staff members are needed to field the many queries, to coordinate the Multicultural and Camino Seguro outreach and services to the Hispanic communities in the state's three grand regions, to update the agency information in the databases, to upgrade the website, and in other ways to manage the many functions of a large, statewide I&R operation.

Beyond increasing in size, Pathfinder improvements also reflect changes over the past two decades in technology and in the state's demographics. When inaugurated in 1997, a phone line and answering machine were sufficient for the staff members to answer queries. But nowadays, many people go to the web for information. Pathfinder staff members have thus created and maintained an up-to-date website programmed to be accessible on smart phones and other devices. Callers can reach Pathfinder through in-person visits, phone calls, e-mails, or the web.

Even more importantly, Pathfinder has evolved in terms of its multicultural outreach. As noted above, the service now employs two Spanish-speaking staff members. In addition to fielding calls and e-mails, these staff members have taken on an outreach function, working with Nashville's Hispanic community—as well as (through Camino Seguro) with the Hispanic communities of Memphis (West Tennessee) and Knoxville and Chattanooga (East Tennessee)—to help Spanish-speaking families. Such help also includes the development of the Camino Seguro website, which serves both families and agencies and is written in English and Spanish. These increased efforts to reach Hispanic families who have members with a disability reflect the increasing Hispanic population in both the Nashville area (over 60,000 individuals, 10% of the city's population) and in the state overall (4.6%, or roughly 300,000 people; Nagle, Gustafson, & Burd, 2012). Pathfinder has also attempted to reach out to Nashville area's Kurdish immigrants. Nashville is home to approximately 12,000 Kurdish immigrants and, as such, has the second largest Kurdish community in North America (Campbell, 2014). As this population has increased over the years, the project has responded by increasing its services to this group. Finally, the products and usage of Pathfinder services have also changed over the years. In earlier days, Pathfinder each year or so produced three phonebook-sized volumes of services for East, Middle, and West Tennessee (respectively). From 2011 on, Pathfinder ceased producing such printed directories.

More recently, Pathfinder staff members have focused on growing and maintaining the web-site. The Camino Seguro portion of the Pathfinder website lists disability and social-service agencies who have Spanish-speaking staff; each listing can be read in English or Spanish by selecting a language choice "button." Through a collaboration with the Tennessee Department of Health, an increased number of social service and health-related agencies have been added to the Pathfinder database. All agencies listed are updated on an annual basis. The Pathfinder Resource Library contains national and Tennessee nonprofit resources that have been reviewed by the Pathfinder staff.

Increasingly, Pathfinder has been able to document, through a REDCap computer-based data entry program, the amounts and locations of Pathfinder requests, along with where such requests came from, types of individuals from whom these requests arose (parents-family members; individuals with disabilities; other agencies), and the specific service(s) requested. In future years, such information will be used to fine-tune Pathfinder's I&R services.

In usage as well, Pathfinder has grown enormously. Given the state's close-knit disability community, increasing numbers of families, individuals, and agency staff have come to hear about Pathfinder and its services. Over time, the Tennessee Disability Pathfinder service has increased its numbers of clients served, from 500–800 in the early 2000s, to approximately 2000 to 2500 in recent years. With better analyses of existing Pathfinder data, one can identify from which areas of the state requests are (and are not) arising, as well as the demographic characteristics of those families requesting specific services (i.e., families whose offspring with disability are of particular ages, disability types, and locations). Using such analyses, future years should see even greater usage of Pathfinder services.

4. THE FUTURE OF DISABILITY-RELATED I&R SYSTEMS

In considering the future of disability-related I&R services, one sees both promises and challenges. Although this mixed picture mirrors that of any I&R service, several promises and challenges seem specific to I&R services that relate to disabilities.

4.1 Promises

Throughout the disability world, a major concern is the degree to which services work together. We thus see mentions of inter-disciplinary, multidisciplinary, and trans-disciplinary teams; of services that are seamless, coordinated, comprehensive, or wrap-around; or that involve one-stop shopping. But though long discussed, disability services remain hard to navigate, with services rarely connected, coordinated, or seamless.

From the perspective of those seeking services, such difficulties arise from multiple directions. At the most basic level, few people outside of disability even know about the local, state, or national disability infrastructure. As shown in Table 1, in every state there exist one or more UCEDDs and multiple agencies of state government that oversee specific disability services; similarly, most states and many localities have parent groups, disability-specific clinics, as well as active chapters of The Arc, Special Olympics, Best Buddies, United Cerebral Palsy, Easterseals, and other organizations. Yet many agencies and organizations are little known to the general public or (at times) even to parents of offspring with disabilities or to the offspring themselves.

Even when aware of a local area's disability services, parents and individuals often find that the system remains difficult to navigate due to the need for specialized knowledge. Consider parents' Special Education rights. Elaborated in federal laws PL 94–142 and IDEA, these rights guarantee to all children a free, appropriate, public education (FAPE), along with the rights of parents to be formally notified about the IEP meeting, to hold that meeting at a time convenient to parents, and to have recourse to an appeal if parents are not satisfied with its outcomes. But as a complicated legal process has now been set in motion, parents find that the IEP meetings are often adversarial, with less knowledgeable, more emotionally invested parents outnumbered by more experienced school personnel. Parents who attempt to learn their rights must drudge through state Special Education procedural safeguards that are written at an average of a 16th grade level—above the reading abilities of many parents (Mandic, Rudd, Hehir, & Acevedo-Garcia, 2012).

Parents report wildly different outcomes in acquiring Special Education services for their children. Although for some parents the process goes smoothly, others feel that they do not receive respect (Wang, Mannan, Poston, Turnbull, & Summers, 2004) and that professionals marginalize them (Turnbull, Turnbull, Erwin, Soodak, & Shogren, 2015). In one study, those parents who were most satisfied with their treatment by the school showed the lowest levels of advocacy activities; in contrast, those with poor experiences with the school were much more likely to bring advocates with them to the meetings, or to learn more about their Special Education rights by talking with other parents, searching the internet, attending workshops, and calling their local Parent Training and Information (PTI) centers (Burke & Hodapp, 2016). In most cases, only after parents had experienced poor treatment (and could not garner appropriate services for their child) did they engage in high levels of advocacy activities.

Partly to address this need for parents to have knowledge of specific service systems, interventions have been developed to train parents and advocates. One such intervention, a 12-week (3-hour/week) workshop series, helps provide parents and advocates an understanding of the IEP process and Special Education rights (Burke, 2013). Another teaches parents about the service system in the immediate post-school years, when parents and their young adult offspring enjoy fewer legal rights in the adult disability system. These workshop series have been shown effective in providing parents of both children and of young adults the knowledge and comfort needed to advocate for services that are difficult to understand and access (Burke et al., 2016; Taylor et al., 2017).

Given this context, disability-related I&R services become essential for families and individuals. Such I&R services unify and coordinate other services, allowing callers to discuss—at once with a single person—the ways that services might go together and how one might approach different agencies and apply for multiple services. I&R service providers can make explicit the many unwritten rules related to eligibility criteria and service delivery. Callers and providers can also explore different potential avenues to receive appropriate services, to address diverse service needs, or to use traditional services in unique ways. In some cases, callers can be referred to experts who are more knowledgeable about a certain type of service. Throughout all these discussions, callers to disability I&R services can be assured that the information that they receive is accurate and up-to-date, that a phone number or email address links to a service organization-agency that currently provides the service being requested.

4.2 Remaining Challenges

Although disability-related I&R services feature many benefits, they have also historically been beset with several challenges. These challenges focus on three main areas.

(1) *Logistical Issues.* Like any ongoing social service, disability-related I&R services need money to begin, grow, and thrive. Start-up costs include paying for employees, housing the service center, and publicizing the service. Although the initial staff may be small—recall that Tennessee Pathfinder began with 1.5 staff members—such paid staff nevertheless requires ongoing financial support. Additional costs accrue when instituting an advertising campaign and when developing databases and websites.

Beyond these initial costs, the financial investment needed for disability I&R services grows as the service expands and becomes increasingly user-friendly. The main costs involve greater numbers of I&R staff, often related to the service expanding to enhance their expertise in a particular area (e.g., adult services), or to reach new geographic areas or families who speak a language other than English. Translating materials into different languages is also expensive. So, too, is it financially challenging to update the database, as that task alone requires time-consuming calls and e-mails to numerous organizations and agencies.

(2) *Utilizing Disability I&R Services to Their Fullest Potentials.* In an early article describing information and referral services, Long (1973) noted that I&R services had two goals. The first, mentioned already, was "to increase the accessibility of human services." The second was "to maximize the utility of information and referral center data for the planning of human services" (Long, 1973, p. 53).

So far when considering disability-related I&R services, this second goal has mostly gone unrealized. Indeed, such services work hard to provide to parents, individuals, and other service agencies the most current, useful information. But disability-related I&R services can also provide snapshots of consumer needs. By better analyzing who calls, about which services, in which localities, one can begin to understand which services are needed by specific groups of individuals with disabilities and their families. Such information might then inform policymakers about how best to deliver services, to target more precisely the recipients of service and the highest-need areas for particular services.

In essence, I&R services may ultimately provide an indirect needs assessment for disability services. In its most general sense, any needs assessment measures "the difference between the current status for the area or topic in consideration (the "*what is*" condition) and its desired status (the "*what should be*" condition)" (Hung & Altschuld, 2013, p. 13). Using this definition, researchers performing needs assessments usually ask a specific group of stakeholders—parents, persons with disabilities, administrators, teachers, or others—to identify needed services. Questions might pertain to identifying those services that are unavailable in a particular area, or that exist but are provided by professionals who have inadequate training, or that only exist if one waits many months or travels long distances. Using such methodologies with parents (and dovetailing parental answers to state board membership and other public data), we have found that in Tennessee behavioral analytic services (provided by Board Certified Behavior

Analysts, or BCBA's) disproportionately exist in or close to the state's main cities (Mello, et al., 2016).

By using data from disability I&R services, however, one can perform needs assessments differently. Instead of asking respondents about the availability and/or quality of each service from a list of disability services, one might identify patterns to the calls or requests themselves. By noting which services are most-often requested and by whom, one can glean a sense of which are most lacking in a particular geographic area, or for individuals of differing ages or with specific disability conditions. Granted, this approach is not perfect. For example, since I&R providers may not ask about each service type individually, some lesser-known services may get missed (e.g., respite care). The numbers of requests for a particular service might therefore not indicate that the service is unavailable, only that its availability is unknown to the caller, which may necessitate more aggressive efforts to make that service known to the public. Still, by examining requested services from disability I&R databases and by dovetailing that information against the numbers of individuals with certain disabilities (e.g., ASD) and of certain ages (e.g., school-children or older adults), in theory one can determine those services most needed in a particular area or by individuals with specific characteristics and their families.

(3) *Becoming a Major Priority to Public-Private Funders.* A final issue concerns the salience and respect of disability I&R services. Recently, we have begun asking knowledgeable individuals across the US whether their states have functioning disability I&R services. Although the picture seems mixed, some respondents have wondered why we are asking. Can't a family or person with disabilities simply go to the web and Google "disability services"? From our perspective, such respondents underestimate the complexity of disability services and how it helps to have a knowledgeable I&R staff member to guide one along the way.

Other issues may also be at play. One wonders whether disability I&R services somehow receive less respect because they are not, strictly speaking, direct services. In this sense, disability I&R services constitute an indirect or even a "meta-"service, more akin to a book's table of contents or index than to its content. Such respondents may perceive disability I&R services as somewhat helpful guides, but not as indispensable services. The perception may even be "Why waste money pointing people to services when you can spend it on the actual services themselves?" Especially given the inadequacy of disability services in most American states, this viewpoint seems understandable.

From our perspective, however, the help provided by disability I&R services constitutes a valuable—even necessary—condition to ultimately accessing disability services. As shown by Table 1, services exist everywhere throughout the U.S., varying by location; individual with disabilities; and other personal, familial, or other conditions. Even the most conscientious, diligent parents or persons with disabilities are unlikely to know about all local services or supports. Unlike a book—which remains unchanged and one can search and re-search again—the specifics of disability services change, are often available for only limited times and for families or individuals with certain qualifications, go under different names, and are offered by different agencies or organizations. In the field of disabilities, there seems a critical need for (disability-specific) I&R services.

5. CONCLUSION

Featuring a long history in the country as a whole, I&R services are only beginning to become prominent in the field of disabilities. As we show in this chapter, the American disability field features many services of different types, even as those services differ by area, by nature of the service provided, by what agency or organization provides the service, and by complicated rules concerning becoming eligible for, applying to, paying for, and accessing a service. Services also change over time, especially those supported by short-term grants or research initiatives. Disability services seem the perfect subject of I&R services.

Our suggestion, then, is that the American disability field follow the country as a whole. Just as the National I&R Triad—the United Way of America (UWA), Administration on Aging (UWA), and the Alliance of Information and Referral Services (AIM)—worked for decades to establish the 2-1-1 information lines that now blanket the country, so, too, can disability communities everywhere work to establish disability-related I&R systems. Once established and publicized, such services can help every family and person with disabilities go beyond hit-or-miss computer searches. By instead utilizing disability-I&R services, parents, individuals, and professionals can attain comprehensive, up-to-date information about how to receive many helpful disability services, regardless of the person's disability, age, financial status, knowledge of the disability community, or where they live.

REFERENCES

Alliance of Information and Referral Systems (AIRS). (2018). *What is I&R? Fairfax*. VA: AIRS. Retrieved from: https://www.airs.org/i4a/pages/index.cfm?pageid=3500.

Association on University Centers on Disabilities. (2012a). *UCEDDs: University centers for excellence in developmental Disabilities: Research, education, service*. Washington, DC: Author.

Association on University Centers on Disabilities. (2012b). *LEND: Leadership education in neurodevelopmental and related Disorders*. Washington, DC: Author.

Berkowitz, E. D. (1980). The politics of mental retardation during the Kennedy administration. *Social Science Quarterly, 61*, 128–143.

Bodie, G. D., Vickery, A. J., Cannava, K., & Jones, S. M. (2015). The role of "active listening" in informal helping conversations: Impact on perceptions of listener helpfulness, sensitivity, and supportiveness and discloser emotional improvement. *Western Journal of Communication, 79*, 151–173.

Burke, M. M. (2013). Improving parental involvement: Training special education advocates. *Journal of Disability Policy Studies, 23*, 225–234.

Burke, M. M., & Hodapp, R. M. (2016). The nature, causes, and correlates of parental advocacy in special education. *Exceptionality: A Special Education Journal, 24*(3), 137–150.

Burke, M. M., Goldman, S. E., Hart, M. S., & Hodapp, R. M. (2016). Evaluating the efficacy of a special education advocacy training program. *Journal of Policy and Practice in Intellectual Disabilities, 13*, 269–276.

Burke, M. M., Patton, K. A., & Lee, C. E. (2016). Parent advocacy across the lifespan. *International Review of Research in Developmental Disabilities, 51*, 193–231.

Campbell, M. (2014). Touring a Kurdish capital in the US. *BBC Magazine—PRI's The World, Aug. 29, 2014*. Retrieved from: http://www.bbc.com/news/magazine-28891241.

Community Ambassadors Providing for Services (CAPS). (2017). *Purpose of information and referral services? Power Point presentation*. Retrieved from: www.capseniors.org.

Coyle, C. E., Putman, M., Kramer, J., & Mutchler, J. E. (2016). The role of Aging and Disability Resource Centers in serving adults aging with intellectual disabilities and their families: Findings from seven states. *Journal of Aging & Social Policy, 28*, 1–14.

Durrance, J. C. (1989). Information needs: Old song, new tune. In , *Proposals for the 1990s: Vol. 2. Rethinking the library* (pp. 159–178). Washington, D.C.: Government Printing Office.

Fujiura, G. T. (2014). The political arithmetic of disability and the American family: A demographic perspective. *Family Relations, 63*, 7–19.

Hatton, C. (2017). Day services and home care for adults with learning disabilities across the UK. *Tizard Learning Disability Review, 22*, 109–115.

Hodapp, R. M., Burke, M. M., Finley, C. I., & Urbano, R. C. (2016). Family caregiving of aging adults with Down syndrome. *Journal of Policy and Practice in Intellectual Disabilities, 13*, 181–189.

Hodapp, R. M., Fidler, D. J., & Depta, E. (2016). Blurring boundaries, continuing change: The next 50 years of research in intellectual and developmental disabilities. *International Review of Research in Developmental Disabilities, 50*, 1–31.

Holl, E., & Meyer, D. (2014). Service system 101: What you need to know about programs for people with intellectual and developmental disabilities (IDD). In D. Meyer, & E. Holl (Eds.), *The sibling survival guide: Indispensable information for brothers and sisters of adults with disabilities* (pp. 93–134). Bethesda, MD: Woodbine House.

Hung, H.-L., & Altschuld, J. W. (2013). Challenges in needs assessment: The Head Start needs assessment national analysis. *Evaluation and Program Planning, 38*, 13–18.

Levinson, R. W. (2002). *New routes to human services: Information and referral*. Springer Series on Social Work. New York: NY: Springer Publishing Company.

Long, N. (1973). Information and referral services: A short history and some recommendations. *Social Service Review, 47*, 49–62.
Magaña, S., Seltzer, M. M., & Krauss, M. W. (2004). The cultural context of caregiving: Differences in well-being between Puerto Rican and non-Latina White mothers of adults with mental retardation. *Mental Retardation, 42*, 1–11.
Mandic, C. G., Rudd, R., Hehir, T., & Acevedo-Garcia, D. (2012). Readability of special education procedural safeguards. *The Journal of Special Education, 45*, 195–203.
Martland, N., & Rothbaum, F. (2006). Thinking critically about the internet: Suggestions for practitioners. *Child Welfare, 85*, 837–852.
Mello, M. P., Goldman, S. E., Urbano, R. C., & Hodapp, R. M. (2016). Services for children with ASD: Comparing rural and non-rural communities. *Education and Training in Autism and Developmental Disorders (ETADD), 51*(4), 355–365.
Nageswaran, S., Parish, S. L., Rose, R. A., & Grady, M. D. (2011). Do children with developmental disabilities and mental health conditions have greater difficulty using health services than children with physical disorders? *Maternal and Child Health Journal, 15*, 634–641.
Nagle, N. N., Gustafson, R., & Burd, C. (2012). *A profile of Hispanic population in the state of Tennessee*. Knoxville, TN: The University of Tennessee Center for Business and Economic Research and Tennessee State Data Center.
National Organization of Rare Diseases (NORD). Rare disease information: NORD's Rare Disease Database. Retrieved from: www.rarediseases.org.
Parish, S. L., Rose, R. A., & Swaine, J. G. (2010). Financial well-being of US parents caring for co-resident children and adults with developmental disabilities: An age cohort analysis. *Journal of Intellectual & Developmental Disability, 35*, 235–243.
Roberts, H., Ingold, A., Liabo, K., Manziotti, G., Reeves, D., & Bradby, H. (2018). Moving on: Transitions out of care for young people with learning disabilities in England and Sweden. *British Journal of Learning Disabilities, 46*, 54–63.
Rogers, C. R. (1957). The necessary and sufficient conditions of therapeutic personality change. *Journal of Consulting Psychology, 21*, 95–103.
Roizen, N. J. (2010). Overview of health issues among persons with Down syndrome. In R. C. Urbano (Ed.), *Vol. 39. International review of research in mental retardation. Special issue on health issues among persons with Down syndrome* (pp. 3–33).
Rubin, R. E. (2004). *Foundations of library and information science* (2nd ed.). New York: Neal-Schuman Publishers, Inc.
Sanderson, K. A., Burke, M. M., Urbano, R. C., Arnold, C. K., & Hodapp, R. M. (2017). Who helps? Characteristics and correlates of informal supporters to adults with disabilities. *American Journal on Intellectual and Developmental Disabilities, 122*, 492–510.
Shorter, E. (2000). *The Kennedy family and the story of mental retardation*. Philadelphia, PA: Temple University Press.
Taylor, J. L., Hodapp, R. M., Burke, M. M., Waitz-Kudla, S. N., & Rabideau, C. (2017). Training parents of youth with autism spectrum disorder to advocate for adult disability services: Results from a pilot randomized controlled trial. *Journal of Autism and Developmental Disorders, 47*, 846–857.
Turnbull, A., Turnbull, R., Erwin, E. J., Soodak, L. C., & Shogren, K. A. (2015). *Families, professionals, and exceptionality: Positive outcomes through partnerships and trust* (7th ed.). Upper Saddle River, NJ: Pearson.
Wang, M., Mannan, H., Poston, D., Turnbull, A. P., & Summers, J. A. (2004). Parents' perceptions of advocacy activities and their impact on family quality of life. *Research and Practice for Persons with Severe Disabilities, 29*, 144–155.
Wark, S., Hussain, R., & Edwards, H. (2014). Impediments to community-based care for people ageing with intellectual disability in rural New South Wales. *Health and Social Care in the Community, 22*, 623–633.

Watanuki, S., Tracy, M. F., & Lindquist, R. (2014). Therapeutic listening. In R. Linquist, M. Snyder, & M. F. Tracy (Eds.), *Complementary and alternative therapies in nursing* (7th ed., pp. 39–53). New York, NY: Springer.

Yan, X.-S. (2011). Information science: Its past, present and future. *Information, 2*, 510–527.

Zaidman-Zait, A., & Jamieson, J. R. (2007). Providing web-based support for families of infants and young children with established disabilities. *Infants & Young Children, 20*, 11–25.

Zigman, W. B. (2013). Atypical aging in Down syndrome. *Developmental Disabilities Research Reviews, 18*, 51–67.